7 Habits to Experience Pain-Free Living!

By

Dr. Derek M. Taylor, D.C.

7 Habits to Experience Pain Free Living!
Copyright © 2017 by Dr. Derek M. Taylor, D.C.

ISBN-13: 978-1546479109

ISBN-10: 1546479104

Dr. Derek M. Taylor, D.C.
Taylor Chiropractic & Laser Center, Inc.
2800 Skypark Drive, Torrance, CA 90505
310-891-0102
doctaylor@torrancepainrelief.com
www.drderektaylor.com

Disclaimer

The information contained in this book is intended for educational purposes only and not intended as medical advice. The author does not assume responsibility or liability for any adverse outcomes resulting directly or indirectly from implementing any advice given in this book. Readers are strongly cautioned to consult a physician or other professional healthcare provider before applying any of the information contained in this book. No book or publication can substitute for professional care or advice.

FORWARD

"My name is Dr. Adam Del Torto, a chiropractor of 31 years and founder of Cranial Facial Release Technique - an advanced form of cranial balloon adjusting, which I teach to other chiropractors. It was at one of my CFR seminars that I first encountered Dr. Derek Taylor.

I could tell right away that he was a very unique individual and a step above the average DC. He impressed me with his inherent knowledge of neurophysiology and specifically cranial function, as he picked up this advanced technique very quickly. Dr. Taylor has since been an active participant in multiple CFR seminars and has greatly contributed with his valuable feedback on how to improve the seminar with recommendations that I immediately incorporated into the course curriculum. For this I am forever grateful.

Shortly after receiving his Advanced CFR Certification, we found ourselves together again at another Cranial Certification Seminar offered by SOTO-USA - a program that was not a required chiropractic curriculum, only attended by the few dedicated and conscientious chiropractors committed to being the best in their profession. Being a chiropractor myself, I get adjusted on a regular basis. Thus, I rarely experience back pain - but for some reason at this seminar my back was acting up and I could barely stand upright. Dr. Taylor pulled me aside and offered to work on me. I was a little hesitant at first, as I am very particular about who I have adjust my spine and am not too confident in most chiropractors' ability, but I was desperate. So Dr. Taylor took charge and started treating me in ways I have never experienced before. His method and approach was so unique, and I can honestly say that with all the myriad of treatments that I have received in the past from other chiropractors - nothing compared to the things that I experienced in that session. I can honestly say that he is one of the best chiropractors I have ever been to, and believe me, I've been to a lot. He is a magician!

If you are looking for a great approach to addressing your symptoms and achieving over all wellbeing, I would highly recommend you read this book - I encourage you to take notes and apply all that you have learned. The information in this book is life-changing, but only if you take action.

One thing I know for sure, EVERYONE should be under the care of a chiropractor, and especially one who is truly loving caring and concerned, and highly competent like Dr. Derek Taylor. His quality of care is unsurpassed and uniquely superior to the vast majority of DC's I have encountered in my 30+ years of being in this great profession. He is the man!"

~Dr. Adam Del Torto, D.C.
Founder of **Cranial Facial Release Technique**

CONTENTS

ACKNOWLEDGEMENTS

This book has been a work in progress over the past 25 years. There are so many people to be thankful for in making this happen.

The first person who comes to mind is the chiropractor who inspired me to become a chiropractor in the first place - Dr. Tim Ursich, D.C. He helped me get out of pain so I was able to play high school football once again.

I'd also like to thank my parents who supported me from kindergarten throughout chiropractic school. Without their support, I don't know what I would've done.

I'm thankful for all the teachers and doctors of chiropractic who have inspired me throughout the years - there are too many to name. Dr. Sheila Laws, D.C. inspired me back in the late 80s when I took her Nimmo Receptor Tonus Method Seminar before I even entered chiropractic school. Dr. Paul Kwik, D.C., for helping me get through chiropractic school by being such a spiritual encouragement to me. My Gonstead mentors – the late Dr. Richard Gohl, D.C., Dr. Kevin Sharp, D.C., Dr. Claudia Anrig, D.C. to name a few. Drs. Paul & Annette Neuman D.C. of Affordable

1

Chiropractic in Ohio, for allowing me to be part of your incredible team of doctors – thank you for giving me a chance and being an incredible blessing to me. Dr. George Roth, D.C., who helped me understand the concept of Matrix Repatterning. The late Dr. Robert Boyd, D.O., who came all the way from Scotland to teach the Bio Cranial Technique. Dr. George Gonzales, D.C., who helped me understand Functional Neurology with the Gonzales Technique. Drs. Scott and Debra Walker, who helped me understand the importance of clearing the Neural Emotional Complex. Dr. Warren Hammer, D.C., for showing me the science behind Adhesive Scar Tissue and using the Graston tools. Dr. Eric Berg, D.C., for teaching me BRT. Dr. Peter Levy, D.C. for teaching me your innovative technique - Neuromuscular Reeducation. Dr. Dan Kalish, D.C. for teaching me how to restore Adrenal Burnout. Dr. Dhatis Karrazzian, D.C. for your brilliance and teaching me about Molecular Mimicry, Autoimmune Disease and Gluten-Sensitivity. Dr. Wally Schmidt, for imparting your 40+ years of experience with Applied Kinesiology- you are a phenomenal doctor. Dr. Adam Del Torto, D.C. for the incredible gift of Craniofacial Release - this technique has been life-changing for some of my patients. Dr. Ted Koren, D.C. who showed me the importance of whole-body adjusting from head to toe, and reminding me of the importance of a Vitalistic Approach.

Please forgive me for not acknowledging all the incredible doctors who have taught me over the years and have made a positive contribution in my life and in the lives of my patients.

Speaking of patients, thank you to all my patients over the years who have taught me so much.

Thank you to my beautiful wife, Alison, who happens to be my most trusted advisor and confidant. Your support and encouragement allows me to keep doing what I'm doing.

To my wonderful children, Hudson, Jonathan, Caden, Dallas, McKenna, Titus, and Jordan, thank you for enriching my life in more ways than you can ever imagine.

Most importantly, I want to thank the Lord for His mercy and grace in my life. Every good and perfect gift has been from Him, and to Him, all I owe.

~Dr. Derek M. Taylor, D.C.

Chapter 1

Could The Pain You're In Really Be Caused By STRESS?

"The doctor of the future will give no medicine
but will interest his patients in the care of the human frame
(spine), in his diet and in the cause and prevention of disease."
~Thomas Edison

"The nervous system controls and coordinates
all of the organs and structures of the human body."
~Grays Anatomy, pg. 4

Every day people come in my office wondering, "Why am I in pain?" It's a good question to ask. In fact, it's a tragedy when people don't ask that question because it tells me they'll probably end up with worse problems in the future. People who aren't asking the question, "Why am I in pain?" end up with greater difficulties because they either ignore or

4

mask the symptom and it usually ends up getting worse over time.

The symptom of pain is your body's way of saying: "There's a problem going on here and you need to get it fixed!" Failure to heed the body's warning signals is like playing Russian roulette. Sometimes the pain may go away for a short period of time. (Be thankful God has given your body an amazing ability to adapt to pain.) Yet sometimes the pain doesn't go away and it gets worse. Your body screams: "You've ignored me long enough so I'm going to make more noise to get your attention!" The pain becomes more intense and more frequent and the next thing you know is…you now suffer with chronic pain.

So let me ask you a question: "Is it easier to fix a problem when it first appears or after it's been there for a long time?" If you're a parent (I happen to fall into this category as a father of seven children) and one of your kids performs an action that's harmful to them or others, you correct them immediately so they won't do it again.

Why immediately?

Because if you don't they'll probably do it again and then…

… the ACTION becomes a HABIT

… the HABIT becomes a CHARACTER TRAIT

… the CHARACTER TRAIT becomes a DESTINY

This is a universal law. Break this law and you end up in big trouble. You can probably think of a few people you know who continue to exhibit traits that may be harmful to themselves and others. Your goal is to not become like them.

Now let me ask you another question: "Is it more expensive to fix a problem when it first appears or after it's been there for a long time?" I'm sure you own a vehicle. When the light on your dashboard says: "Service Engine Soon," do you take your car into the service station immediately or do you wait two years and then take it in? Of course you take it in immediately because if you don't, the problem can become more complicated and get worse; now it's going to cost you A LOT MORE MONEY to fix. Those who are wise get their oil changed every 3,000 miles, tires rotated every 5,000 miles, and the recommended service updates at the appointed times because it COSTS LESS MONEY to MAINTAIN than to REPAIR.

This is why it's EXTREMELY IMPORTANT to ask the question: "Why am I in pain?" Ignoring or masking the pain results in FUTURE PROBLEMS. And you don't want future problems. You want solutions today. You want to AVOID future problems and the first step is to understand what causes the pain. When patients come into my office wanting to get rid of their pain, I'm happy they're there. It tells me they're asking the question: "Why am I in pain?" They're THINKING. They're ASKING QUESTIONS. They're PROACTIVE. This is a good thing! This is the first step in their journey to LIVING PAIN-FREE.

Now the next thing you need to know is that most people don't know the REAL reason they're dealing with their pain. They think they have an idea but it's usually wrong. So-and-so told him "this" is the cause, or that doctor said "this" is the cause, or the Internet said "this" is the cause. And so they chase "the alleged cause" of their pain with no results because they're trying to solve the wrong problem. They're barking up the wrong tree. They're climbing up a ladder that's leaning against the wrong wall.

So what is most likely the REAL cause of your pain? The answer is probably simple…. STRESS! (Understand that sometimes pain may be caused by a serious medical condition, but this is more the exception rather than the rule.)

STRESS is the Cause! STRESS is the reason why you are in pain! That's it, pure and simple! Research shows that over 80% of all health problems are caused by some form of stress. What I refer to as "the three secrets" are actually three types of stress: #1 PHYSICAL STRESS, #2 CHEMICAL STRESS, and #3 EMOTIONAL STRESS.

Any one of these stressors can cause your pain. And it's usually a combination of all three that bring about the symptoms of pain. The key is discovering the MAIN stressor that's causing your pain. Identifying the main source of stress and making the necessary corrections often provides immediate relief. If you stress something, either forcefully or long enough, it WILL break. Imagine a 2" x 4" thick board about 6 feet long laid out across on two sawhorses. Without any stresses placed on this board, it can lay there forever without any change or damage to it. Now what would happen if I place a 10 pound weight in the center of the board? The board will slightly bend because of the stress placed on it. If I continue to increase the weight, the board continues to bend more to the point that it breaks. This is what happens with your body, stress is placed on it until it finally 'breaks' and then pain appears. Understand that when stress occurs in your life, whether it's physical, chemical, or emotional stress, it causes wear and tear which eventually leads to a breakdown, which typically manifests in some type of pain.

So why are you in pain? The answer is STRESS…Physical stress, chemical stress, emotional stress, or typically a combination of the three.

In this chapter, I would like to go into detail explaining the concept of physical stress. Physical stress can be defined as stress to the body, primarily the structural frame in the form of the bones and muscles, but more importantly the nervous system.

The nervous system is the most important system in the body. Why? Because it was the very first bodily system formed and it controls every cell, tissue, organ, and system of the body. The nervous system is so important that it's the only system totally encased by bone. Its primary components are the brain which is encased by the cranial vault and the spinal cord which is protected by the bones in your spinal column.

Let's talk about the structural imbalances that can negatively affect the nervous system. Here are the primary areas or issues that can physically put stress on your nervous system:

- the bones in your spine (vertebral subluxations)
- the bones in your skull (facial & cranial bone misalignments)
- dropped arches in the feet (pronated feet)
- adhesive scar tissue build-up in the muscles
- poor posture
- incorrect exercises not appropriate for your body
- incorrect mechanics in activities of daily living
- unsupportive shoes
- untreated old injuries
- a poor, unsupportive mattress
- anything that you're doing on a daily basis that distresses tissues beyond their limits

When the nerves exit from the spinal cord, they can be damaged by a misaligned vertebra; this is what's called a subluxation and is the primary reason people see a chiropractor. Hard bone on a soft nerve causes pain. Vertebral subluxations lead to joint restrictions. Lack of movement leads to inflammation and toxic build-up in the surrounding joints. In addition, when the nerves are irritated, choked, or pinched the surrounding musculature goes into spasm and adhesive scar tissue forms in the muscle. Adhesive scar tissue not only leads to pain in that particular muscle, but it can also refer pain to different areas of the body.

Failure to properly address the adhesive scar tissue is often why people can't get rid of their pain. What I've discovered is the pain isn't often coming from the place you think it's coming from. For example, I recently treated a woman who experienced excruciating pain in her lower back. However, the source of her pain was coming from her psoas major muscle, which is a hip flexor muscle on the front of the body. When we reduced the adhesive scar tissue in this muscle her pain immediately went away. I see this every day in my practice. The pain is in one area of the body, but the source is coming from an unrelated area.

Another commonly overlooked physical stress is put on the brain by misaligned cranial bones. About 20% of your nervous system passes through your spine; yet 80% is in the cranium. The brain is the most important part of your nervous system and if your nervous system controls and coordinates every cell, tissue, organ, and system of the body, then it's important that your brain is functioning at its peak. For years I only focused on the 20% of the nervous system in the spine. Recently, however, I've been focusing more on the other 80% and I'm excited to see the changes that occur in the body when the brain functions optimally.

Headaches, sinus problems, breathing problems, thyroid dysfunction, stomach problems, back problems, and pain anywhere in the body can be caused by stress on the nervous system. It's essential that your nervous system is functioning properly and free from any interference caused by cranial bones and vertebra being out of alignment.

Here's a simple way to determine if your cranial bones and spinal vertebrae are in alignment. Stand in front of a full length mirror and observe your posture. Use this checklist to determine if you're in alignment:
*Look at your pant/belt line. Is it parallel with the floor or is one side tilted higher?
*Look at your shoulder level. Is it balanced or is one side tilted higher?
*Look at your ear level. Is it balanced or is one side tilted higher?

*Look at your eye level. Are your eyes evenly balanced or is one eye tilted higher?

If you're tilted on any of these levels, your nervous system will be stressed and won't function at optimal levels.

Keep in mind that your nervous system is much more complex than what I've described in this chapter. So make sure you get regular checkups with a practitioner who looks at the whole person and corrects the structural imbalances located throughout your entire body.

In Chapters 3-9 I'll give you 7 habits to decrease the three types of stress: physical, chemical, and emotional, but first I would like to share the secret to recovering quickly from pain or any health challenge you may be facing.

"My son, Matthew, broke his leg in a bicycle accident on August 23, 2016, snapping his femur in half. The next day, he had major surgery with a titanium rod placed in the femur to repair it. The Orthopedic Surgeon said that the soonest he would be able to play a sport again would be in January or February, but he probably wouldn't be very good at it. He said it would take about a full year to recover from the injury before he would play like himself again. A week after the surgery, he was still in a wheelchair and could barely stand up without being nauseated and throwing up.

Matthew was not cleared by the Orthopedic Surgeons office to go to school for the month of September. I took Matthew to see Dr. Taylor who said he could help speed up the recovery using his methods and technology. He laid out a treatment plan for Matthew and he started treatments right away. Matthew noticed significant improvements with Dr. Taylor's treatments from day one and he continued to get better after every visit. When Matthew went back for a follow up visit a few weeks later at the Orthopedic Surgeons office, the Surgeon looked at us in disbelief when he discovered that Matthew got out of his chair and sat on the table without pain. He couldn't believe he was not on pain meds. He did an evaluation and Matthew was cleared to go back to school and play sports again including football. The first practice of flag football, he did well. The following week he started as quarterback. Eight weeks later he led his team to the championship game. Thanks to Dr. Taylor, with all his technology, research and knowledge, my son went from a broken femur with a titanium rod in a wheelchair with no hope to playing football in four weeks and leading his team to win the division championship." ~Robert Espinoza

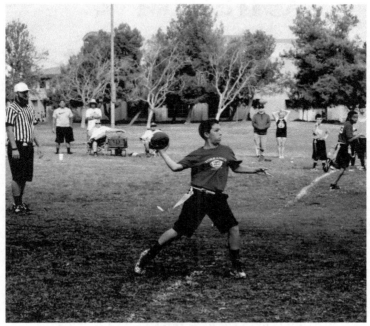

(Matthew Espinosa)

Chapter 2

The Secret To Recovering Quickly From Pain

"All trials are not the reason to give up, but a challenge to improve ourselves. Our pain is not an excuse to back out, but an inspiration to move on."
~Unknown

"When it is dark enough, you can see the stars."
~Ralph Waldo Emerson

Have you ever wondered why sometimes you have a pain that is short-lived, and other times the pain is there constantly and doesn't seem to be going away? Why does this happen? The answer can be found in one word...TIME. It typically goes like this... The longer you've had the pain, the longer time it takes to get rid of it. The shorter you've had the pain, the shorter time it takes to get rid of it. For example, this past week I treated two different patients who were in two different car accidents. "Patient A" experienced her car accident six months ago and was in pain all that time before coming to see me. "Patient B" experienced her car accident a week ago and came to see me the day of the accident. After three visits, can you guess which patient is almost pain free? Yes, you guessed right... "Patient B."

On the contrary, after nine visits, "Patient A" is still in quite a bit of pain. Does this mean that the pain will never go away? No, it just means it is going to take more time. The problem is MORE COMPLEX. Pain is your body's way of telling you there is a problem somewhere and it needs to be corrected. If you fail to correct the problem, your body will compensate and compromise other areas of your body, and now the simple problem becomes a complex one. Complex problems are much more difficult to treat, take more time, and costs more money. Simple problems are much easier to treat, take less time, and costs less money. Recently, I took one of our vehicles to the shop for a checkup. The mechanic said he discovered oil leaking from the drive axle with a few bearings missing. I asked him, "Is it safe to drive the car in this condition?" He said, "Yes, you can drive it like this for another six months to a year, but you will eventually want to get it fixed because when this joint is not working properly, the other surrounding areas will wear out quicker and it will end up costing you more money." I really didn't FEEL like paying $1,200 to fix a problem that wasn't urgent, but I GLADLY made the investment because I didn't want to pay $2,500 a year from now for a problem that would be more complex.

So here's the take away. The sooner you TAKE ACTION with a problem, the sooner you RESOLVE the problem. Don't let your problems cause more problems for you by not taking action. Don't settle for the STATUS QUO because you figured it just has to be this way.
Taking fast action is critical for getting rid of pain quickly.

You may be wondering, what if I never took action with my pain and I'm in a state of chronic pain, what do I do now? Well, like I mentioned above, it will be more difficult and challenging to get rid of the pain, but that doesn't mean you will always have to live with pain. Relief can still be found that is long-lasting, effective, and complete.

So the next thing you need to understand is that it is very important to know where the pain came from in the first place, what steps you need to take to get rid of it, and what realistic time frame you're looking at before it will go away. As I mentioned in the previous chapter the cause of the pain is due to stress: physical stress, chemical stress, and emotional stress.

You get rid of the pain by getting rid of the stress. The sooner you understand this concept, the faster you'll heal and the sooner the pain will go away. I like to make the analogy that your health is like your personal checking account. Whenever you're exposed to some sort of stress— whether physical, chemical, or emotional—it's like making a withdrawal from your checking account.

The more withdrawals you have, the weaker, sicker, and more painful your body becomes. The concept is simple: if you're constantly making withdrawals from your checking account, you need to put in deposits to replenish your account. Too many withdrawals without enough deposits will lead to an empty bank account with creditors knocking on your door wanting to be paid.

The same is true when it comes to our health. Too often, we overload our lives with stressors that act as withdrawals to our health account.

It's a very simple concept: if you have more withdrawals than deposits, you're in the negative and that's bad. If you have more deposits than withdrawals, you're in the positive and that's good! This is not rocket science but common sense. We all accumulate stress over our lifetime. We're constantly withdrawing from our health account and not replenishing it with deposits. If you do this over a period of time it's not long before you're deep in debt.

People clearly understand that taking money out of their bank account without replenishing it with deposits will soon cause financial problems for them. However, they fail to understand that the stresses of life take away from their health like a withdrawal does on their bank account and they don't continue to add deposits that will replenish their health like a deposit does on their bank account.

Over time, the withdrawals from stress starts to add up until the accumulated effect starts to wreak havoc on their health and that's typically when the pain or other symptom begins to manifest. The pain or symptom is usually an annoyance at first, so it is ignored, but then it becomes more intense as their body is trying to tell them that there is a problem that needs to be addressed. By the time people reach my office, their body is SCREAMING at them for help and the accumulated effect of stress takes more time to unwind and correct.

You must make daily health deposits that will strengthen your body and mind to counteract the constant stresses you face each day if you want to experience optimal health and pain-free living.

The remainder of this book is all about the daily deposits you can make to counteract the daily stresses of life and if you follow the principles I am about to give you, it will be life-changing.

The remaining chapters answer the questions my patients have been asking me for the past 25 years:

"What can I do to help myself get better?"

"What can I do to speed up the healing process?"

"What can I do to prevent the pain/problem from coming back?"

"Now that I've regained my health, what can I do to maintain what I've achieved?"

I've boiled down the key components that keep you healthy physically, chemically and mentally/emotionally. Incorporate these 7 habits that you will be learning in the following chapters and you'll not only be placing deposits in your account to decrease your pain, but improve the overall quality and longevity of your health like you've never seen before.

"I came to see Dr. Taylor for an autoimmune condition that was causing severe pain in my left eye. I went to different practitioners for help but found no relief. One practitioner put me on a supplement that caused me to have a severe reaction that sent me to the emergency room. I had to have shots directly in my eye to save it from being lost. I had seen Dr. Taylor years ago but moved and was no longer under his care. After this episode of pain I decided to give him a call and get back under his care. He immediately identified the problem and got me on a course of treatment to resolve my autoimmune condition. After three months of care, I was a new person. The pain in my eye is completely gone and I have not had a single episode of pain in over a year. He not

only takes care of me, but also my husband and children."
~Katie Donaho

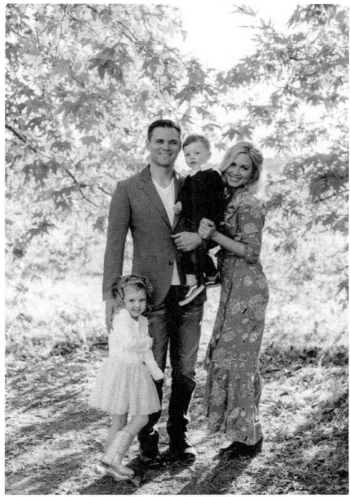

(The Donaho Family)

Chapter 3

Feel Great NOW: What You Should & Shouldn't EAT

"Let food be thy medicine and medicine be thy food."
~Hippocrates, Father of Modern Medicine

"Those who think they have no time for healthy eating,
will sooner or later have to find time for illness."
~Edward Stanley

"Your body doesn't have the ability to turn garbage into a high
quality product. All of your cells, muscles, skin bones, etc.
are built by the food that you supply. Choose wisely."
~Unknown

Over 100 million adults in the United States suffer with chronic pain every day, which exceeds the total number of people impacted by diabetes, heart disease, and cancer.

Many of these cases do not have an initial injury or disease associated with the pain, which leaves the underlying cause of pain a total mystery.

Q: What can be causing this mysterious pain or symptom?

A: The food and/or beverages they are consuming on a daily basis.

Here's my point: if you're dealing with a symptom or an unresolved problem that you haven't been able to solve, the problem may be caused by something you're eating or drinking every day.

If you eat something that your body considers to be bad, you're going to feel bad—somewhere in the body. In other words, if you eat something your body doesn't agree with, it will create a symptom somewhere in your body. Sometimes the symptoms are obvious, other times they're not.

How does the food I eat influence my symptoms or pain levels?

You may have a food allergy or food sensitivity that is creating an immune response, which leads to inflammation and therefore pain.

The difference between a food allergy and a food sensitivity is that the food allergy typically triggers an immediate antibody reaction and you experience the symptom right away. Food sensitivities, on the other hand, trigger slower response in the cells and sometimes may not show up until the next day or even later. Food allergies have obvious symptoms. Food sensitivities are more subtle and disguised.

Food allergies and sensitivities not only can cause pain in the body, but a host of other symptoms that people do not associate their influence with side effects including:

- ✓ Headaches
- ✓ Brain fog
- ✓ Belly Fat
- ✓ Chronic Cough
- ✓ Learning Disorders
- ✓ Sore Throat
- ✓ Anxiety
- ✓ Depression
- ✓ Skin Disorders
- ✓ Weakened Vision
- ✓ ADHD
- ✓ Excessive Anger
- ✓ Earache…and the list goes on…

These are just a few symptoms. You need to understand that any symptom in the body can be caused by a food sensitivity that you are completely unaware of and don't even know you have.

What are the most common foods that people are allergic or sensitive to that I should stay away from?

#1) Gluten: This is the protein found in wheat, barley, rye, spelt, and triticale. If you just eliminate this one food item from your diet, you'll pay big dividends for your health. Even if you don't think you're gluten sensitive, understand that if you're of British, Irish, Scottish, Eastern European, Scandinavian, or Jewish ancestry you should stay away from gluten. Why? Because you're more susceptible to gluten sensitivity and thus an autoimmune disease such as Hashimoto's Thyroiditis, Diabetes, Connective Tissue Disorders, Alzheimer's, and more. This one food item can cause a symptom anywhere in your body, including your mind. It's best if you stay away from it altogether. On another note, just because something is labeled "gluten-free," doesn't mean it's good for you as it can have a high sugar content, such as in some gluten-free breads. I've even seen the "gluten-free" label on products that aren't even grain-related like drinks, so read labels carefully! In addition, it is advisable to not only be tested for sensitivities to oats, corn, brown rice, and quinoa, but stay entirely away from these grains as well. Although these foods do not contain gluten, they may be a cross-reactive food that can cause pain and inflammation in your body.

#2) Casein: This is the protein found in dairy products such as cow's milk and even goat's milk. In fact, this protein is found in all animal milk except for camels. Casein is in the common foods most of us eat and love like cheese, yogurt (including frozen yogurt), ice cream, and of course milk. Regular consumption can flare up Irritable Bowel Syndrome, Respiratory and Sinus Disorders, Skin Disorders, and it has even been linked to Type 1 Diabetes in children. Most people do not digest dairy well, with the exception of the following races of people: English, German, Austrian, Finnish, and French. However, this doesn't mean if you're of one of these races it's perfectly fine to eat dairy. Organic Butter & Ghee (clarified butter) are processed differently and most of my patients do not have a problem consuming them.

#3) GMO: Genetically Modified Organisms are living organisms whose genetic material has been artificially manipulated in a laboratory through genetic engineering. This science creates unstable combinations of plant, animal, bacteria, and viral genes that don't occur naturally. The reason food is genetically modified is to produce increased yields, enhanced nutrition, and pesticide tolerance; however this is often not the case. Genetically modified food is most common in refined carbohydrates. Although gluten isn't found in the molecular structure of corn, oats, quinoa, and amaranth, these foods are often genetically modified or cross contaminated with gluten. So if you eat corn, for example, make sure it's non-GMO and organic. If you're not sure how your body will do with these foods you can always do the indicator testing to see how your body does with them. Current research has connected GMOs with health problems, environmental damage, and the violation of farmers' as well as consumers' rights. Stay away from GMO foods.

Here are some other foods that may not cause allergies or sensitivities, but they can cause inflammation and pain in the body:

#1) Sugar: White sugar, brown sugar, and everything that ends with "ose" including fructose and sucrose is considered a sugar. This also includes agave nectar, honey, and maple syrup. Sugar is addicting. Especially stay clear of anything that has high fructose corn syrup, which is in more foods than you can imagine. Understand that the corn used in high fructose corn syrup is probably GMO so that's another reason to eliminate it from your diet. Sugar has a stimulating effect on the cells in your brain and makes you crave more, especially if you have a thyroid problem. I once found a list of over 100 illnesses that can be linked to sugar, so there's no need for it in a healthy lifestyle.

#2) Saturated Fats/Trans Fats: These increase bad cholesterol and are found in fried foods, fast foods, commercially baked goods, and foods prepared with partially hydrogenated oil, margarine, and most vegetable oils. Also, watch out for common cooking oils like safflower, soy, sunflower, corn, and canola oil. These fats can have a high content of Omega-6 fatty acids, which affect your anti-inflammatory producing Omega-3 fatty acids.

#3) Chemical Additives/Preservatives: The biggest offenders are MSG (Monosodium Glutamate) and

Aspartame. These have excitotoxins and neurotoxins which damage the brain and cause the body to react with inflammation. These additives are not natural and your body has difficultly processing them. MSG has been a major hidden cause of headaches for my patients. I've seen it cause joint pain and swelling in the joints, especially the fingers, wrists, knees, and feet. Additionally steer clear of Sodium Sulfite, Sodium Nitrate, Sodium Nitrite, BHA, BHT, and other ingredients you're not familiar with. They're all man-made chemicals that supposedly preserve for a longer shelf life and enhance the flavor of food, but instead cause havoc in your body which is not designed to process anything artificial. You'll find additives and preservatives in any foods that are processed, packaged, and refined—which generally come in boxes and cans. The white salt that's been added has been heated, crushed, and run through nickel plates. This form of salt is unable to be digested because the sodium chloride bond has been welded together, thus raising your blood pressure and creating inflammation.

#4) Alcohol: Especially watch out for alcoholic beverages made from gluten-containing grains like you find in beer. Alcohol, when consumed in excess—which is more than two drinks a day— is a major stressor to the liver, pancreas, and fat tissue in the body. Since alcohol is a refined sugar, it's rapidly absorbed and is toxic to nerve tissue. Alcohol needs to be detoxified by the liver to be eliminated, but overconsumption impedes the liver's ability to eliminate the alcohol. If you're going to drink at all, a better choice would be gluten-free vodka or tequila (which is made from cactus). But still limit yourself to no more than two drinks per day!

#5) Feedlot-Raised Meat: Animals such as cows, pigs, and fowl that are fed GMO grains like soy and corn will create high inflammation in your body when you eat them. The fat from the feedlot-raised meat is high in a substance called arachidonic acid which triggers inflammation. This meat also contains hormones, antibiotics, and other xeno-estrogens that are inflammatory in humans.

#6) Advanced Glycation End Products: AGEs are harmful compounds that stem from cooking protein or fat at high temperatures with sugar. Have you ever barbecued chicken or beef with teriyaki sauce and it formed that glazed, caked coating over the meat? That's glycation and it's deadly for the body. This is a hidden source of chronic inflammation that most people don't know about. It has also been linked to Type 2 Diabetes, Cardiovascular Disease, and Premature

Aging, as it causes the cells in your body to stiffen and become less pliable. Have you ever seen a burnt piece of barbecued teriyaki beef? It's stiff as a board. That piece of meat is doing the same thing to the cells inside of your body when you eat it.

How do I discover which foods are creating inflammation, pain, or some other symptom in my body?

A common way of determining which foods are harmful to you is to use a food diary. Simply record everything you consume from the time you wake up, to the time you go to bed including all food foods, beverages, snacks, even vitamins, medications, and personal care products (remember anything you put on the skin is absorbed and transported into your body). Record how you feel after you consume something. Typically, the foods we are most sensitive to are foods that we are consuming on a daily basis. It is not uncommon for these foods to be something that we crave and would never consider giving up, as they can have an addictive property to them. Once you have a suspect food, eliminate that from your diet for 2 weeks and then see how you feel during that period of time. You will typically feel better unless you are also consuming something else that you're not aware of that is causing you to have problems. After the 2 week period of time, reintroduce the food by itself and see how you feel. You will most likely feel bad shortly after consuming it.

"Your body keeps an accurate journal regardless of what you write down."

~Unknown

If you do this process and you still can't figure out which foods are causing the problem, you can also do a pulse test. Here are the steps to perform a pulse test:

1) Take your pulse by placing your three middle fingers over your wrist on the thumb side (do not use your thumb as it has its own pulse) for one whole minute and record the number.

2) Eat a food that you suspect is causing you to have problems.

3) Take your pulse again for one whole minute, 20 minutes after consuming this food. (Make sure you eat the food by itself and it is not combined with another ingredient as it can give you a false reading.)

4) If your pulse either goes up or down six beats after eating the food, you most likely have an allergy or sensitivity to it.

5) Eliminate this food from your diet.

If you're still not sure which food is causing you to have problems after doing these two methods, I recommend you do food sensitivity testing with a trained practitioner who can pinpoint your problem with accuracy. I use muscle response testing at our office to determine which foods are causing you to have a problem and can pinpoint with accuracy these sensitivities in about 15 minutes. I've seen lives changed as a result of my patients changing their diet and symptoms that people struggled with for years vanish over a 3-4 week period of time after changing their diet.

Once my patients discover which foods they should not be eating, they always ask me…

"Which foods should I be eating?"
Here's a short list of anti-inflammatory foods that I recommend consuming on a regular basis:

#1) Organic Vegetables and Fruits: Since there are more than 500 different chemicals routinely used on conventional produce, eating organic is a no-brainer. It's preferable if you eat your veggies raw or lightly steamed, as cooking kills nutrients and the raw enzymes in vegetables that are essential for digestion. All vegetables are fine; however, regarding fruit, stick to those below 55 on the glycemic index such as berries and citrus to avoid excess sugar in your diet.

#2) Organic Chicken, Turkey, and Eggs: Organic fowl are much healthier than conventional poultry because they're not injected with antibiotics and hormones. Eat eggs that are organic, free-range, and Omega-3 enriched since they are lower in arachidonic acid which causes inflammation.

#3) Wild-Caught Fish: Wild-caught fish like salmon and tuna are higher in healthy Omega-3 fatty acids and are significantly higher in DHA (Docosahexaenoic Acid) and EPA (Eicosapentaenoic Acid) which are excellent "brain foods" and wonderful for decreasing inflammation.

#4) Limited Grains and Legumes: Rice, quinoa, and lentils, among other grains and legumes, are to be used sparingly.

#5) Healthy Fats: When you think of healthy fats to eat, think of the pneumonic **B-A-C-O-N**:

*B*utter, *A*vocados, *C*oconut oil, *O*live oil, *N*uts

In addition to foods, I must also mention environmental toxins and allergens that can sabotage your health, such as household cleaning products, plastic containers/products that are touching your food, fire retardants on your furniture/clothes, chemicals saturated in new building materials, dust, and molds. You need to pay attention to these factors as well as your diet. For example, I had a patient who always felt weak and sick at home, but felt great whenever she spent time outside the home. She discovered a hidden mold in her house that was causing her immune system to weaken and create inflammation which caused pain.

Pain can also be caused by toxic dental material that is leaking from the tooth into your body. It is well known that Mercury fillings are toxic, but most people do not understand the importance of using biocompatible material with your teeth. My Dentist, Dr. Glenn Sperbeck, D.D.S., uses specific dental materials that are biocompatible with your body. Having material in your teeth that your body does not agree with can create health challenges as your healthy tissue rejects the incompatible material.

I've also seen patients on certain prescription medications where the side effects from the medication caused pain. Read the side effects to the prescription medication if you're taking any, and consider whether or not it may be causing pain somewhere in the body. If this is the case, talk with your medical doctor about possibly switching to a different medication that may be more compatible with your body. Now that you're aware of the physical and chemical stresses that may be causing your pain, we'll next examine the final stressor: your emotions, which is an all too common form of stress!

"I was experiencing severe pain in my neck and back as a result of being in a bad car accident. In addition, the accident was causing me to have constant headaches that I experienced on a daily basis. Dr. Taylor's treatments brought immediate relief. However, the headaches persisted

and wouldn't go away. Dr. Taylor did some food testing on me and discovered I was allergic to corn as well as a few other foods I wasn't aware of. As soon as I made the change in my diet, the headaches got better and better until they were GONE. This was a BIG GAME CHANGER for me and my overall health. Also, a year later, my husband and I were able to conceive and have a beautiful baby girl. I believe making the change in my diet led me to be healthier and more fertile." ~Caitlin Baitzel

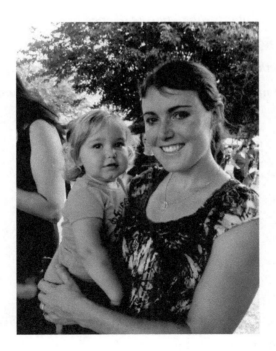

(Caitlin Baitzel & daughter)

Chapter 4

Stop EMOTIONS From Manifesting In Your Body!

"A man's mind may be likened to a garden,
which may be intelligently cultivated or allowed to run wild;
but whether cultivated or neglected, it must, and will, bring
forth. If no useful seeds are put into it, then an abundance of
useless weed seeds will fall therein,
and will continue to produce their kind."
~ James Allen

"As a man thinketh in his heart, so is he."
~ Proverbs 23:7

Most people do not understand the important concept that emotional stress and trauma can be a major source of pain. 80% of all primary health care physician visits are associated with emotional stress. The problem with stress is that most people think it only affects your mental or emotional state and they fail to make the connection that stress affects the body.

Let's say, for example, you are worrying about a situation you feel you have no control over; there are no solutions to the problem, the problem only seems to be getting worse; and on top of that, no one knows that you are struggling with this issue because you have kept all this to yourself.

Your body will release stress hormones such as norepinephrine, epinephrine, and cortisol which prepares you to physically run from the situation. Blood flow is immediately shut down to your gastrointestinal tract. What does that cause? A decrease in the release of hydrochloric acid and digestive enzymes to break down your food. This leads to poor digestion, acid reflux, and pain in the stomach area. When the stomach is inflamed and stressed, it often refers pain to the neck and middle back. Blood flow will also be decreased to the pancreas. This affects your ability to release insulin and failure to have adequate amounts of insulin in your blood leads to diabetes. Poor blood flow to the pancreas will also stress this organ and stress to the pancreas can refer pain to the left shoulder blade and middle back. Blood flow also is decreased to the brain which leads to inability to concentrate and think properly. Brain fog, poor decision-making, and forgetfulness become the norm, which leads to more anxiety and a decreased quality of life. Chronic lack of blood flow to the brain caused the brain cells to die which can lead to dementia and Alzheimer's disease.

What about the muscles? Blood flow is INCREASED so you are rearing to go and run away from your situation. However, when you don't use those muscles (*this is why it's important to exercise on a regular basis and why you feel better after exercising...because you've just released accumulated stress and energy stored in the muscles and other hormones are released to relax you*) metabolites and waste products from the un-used energy gets stored in the muscles, and toxins accumulate leading to tight and tender muscle fibers which leads to pain. If you ever try to give a massage to somebody who has been stressed for a long period of time, you will see that most of them cannot handle much pressure as it is too painful to the touch. This is especially the case of they have a poor diet and are eating processed foods, sugar, and all the junk that they reach for when they are stressed. These are just a few examples of how the body is affected by emotional stress. Understand that any organ or part of the body can be affected by stress including the heart, lungs, liver, kidneys, adrenals, reproductive organs, thyroid, and the list goes on.

What should I NOT do when I am experiencing emotional stress?

I mentioned earlier that emotional stress will release hormones to prepare your body to fight or run from your situation. Fuel is required to make this happen. Most people will turn to a quick source of fuel in the form of glucose or sugar such as bread, pasta, chips, cookies, ice cream, sodas, bobas, beer, wine, cocktails, pastries, 'protein bars,' etc. While they are snacking on their 'fix,' they will turn on the TV set to take their mind off the problem, such as the news or some 'high adrenaline' action movie to 'relax' them. This is not good, as it only adds fuel to the fire, making the problem worse. However, the biggest mistake I see in my practice when someone is struggling emotionally with the challenges of everyday life is ... DOING NOTHING! In other words, ignoring the stress, burying the stress, or pretending the stress is not there. Let's face it, we all have struggles and challenges we face on a daily basis. How you handle the stresses in your life will have a HUGE impact on your overall health. The point I want you to understand is that you need a way of releasing the emotional stressors you are dealing with instead of just holding them in and ignoring them. It takes energy to hold on to emotional stressors - energy that could be used for your activities of daily living, focusing on your current tasks, or even healing. Holding on to emotional stress is like trying to hold an inflated beach ball underneath the surface of the water. It takes energy to keep that ball underneath the surface. However, when you let go of the ball, there is a sense of relief as you are no longer struggling with the ball.

I understand that releasing emotional stress is not an easy thing to do. Most people find it extremely uncomfortable to confront the emotional challenges they are experiencing on a daily basis. In fact, day after day, week after week, month after month, and year after year when emotions are not dealt with, your body can actually create a physical pain to distract you from dealing with the deeper emotional struggles that you have ignored. Confronting the emotional pain you are experiencing can be so difficult and challenging for your body to handle, that pain can develop anywhere in the body as a means to keep you from dealing with your emotional struggles. Have you ever had a pain that was chronic or lasted longer than you expected, and then one day it suddenly disappears? What happened? Often times, the cure was dealing with that emotional struggle inadvertently and the body no longer needed to create a pain as a diversion.

This can be a very difficult concept to grasp, especially in light of the fact that most people want to ignore their emotional struggles altogether.

Getting to the root cause of the patient's emotional challenges is probably the most difficult aspect of my practice. Why? Because most people would rather not go down the path of releasing past hurts, anxieties, and fears.

In addition, when pain becomes a source of distraction, the patient has another challenge of always focusing on the pain. What I see in my office is that patients are constantly focusing on their pain. They tell themselves, "I have pain in my_____" (fill in the blank) and they are reinforcing the problem in their brain. They also talk about their pain with other people which also reinforces pain in that area. If they would just focus on releasing any emotional stressors they are dealing with, it could have a profound impact on reducing the pain. It is also beneficial not to talk about the pain as if it is a regular part of your life. I'm not trying to minimize when a person is dealing with a real issue of pain. My point is that constant attention and focus on pain can perpetuate the pain for weeks, months, years, and even decades.

How Do I Eliminate the Mental/Emotional Stress?

Our tendency is to avoid pain! Dealing with your emotions can often times be painful. If you don't relate on the emotional level, there's less chance of being hurt. However, if you can learn how to deal with your emotions in an effective and healthy manner, it can greatly reduce your stress levels, and thus, decrease your pain and improve your health. So how do you move towards relating on an emotional level that will help you decrease pain levels and increase your health?

First you need to understand that failure to express your emotions can lead to increased stress, decreased health, and increased pain. Humans were designed to express emotions in a healthy way. Failure to do so creates problems, such as pain. Next, understand that your natural bent is to NOT share on an emotional level. It can be painful or uncomfortable, and it's much easier to travel down the path of least resistance. Thirdly, you can actually develop a pain somewhere in your body as a means to distract you from having to deal with a negative emotion you're experiencing such as anger or sadness. Your brain can create pain somewhere in your body to keep the negative emotion buried in your subconscious mind. (*Realize that we label these emotions as "negative," while they're only normal emotions on the emotional spectrum. We all experience sadness, anger, and fear, just as we experience joy, peace, and contentment. However, the primary emotions humans struggle with are anger and anxiety, which most of us consider to be negative*).

I've found that in my 25 years of practice, failure to understand and embrace these three fundamental concepts about emotions will make it very difficult or almost impossible for someone to get out of chronic pain—if the emotional component is the biggest source of stress. It's not that these people can't be helped at all; it's just that their healing and results will be limited.

If, however, you are willing to understand and embrace these essential components to emotional health, here's what you

47

can do to decrease the emotional/mental stress in your life that may be contributing to your pain:

#1) Review these three factors mentioned above:

A) Failure to express your emotions can lead to increased stress, decreased health, and increased pain.

B) Your natural bent is NOT to share on an emotional level.

C) You can develop pain in your body as a means to distract you from having to deal with the negative emotion you're experiencing.

#2) Identify the PROBLEM & the EMOTION associated with the problem. Then work towards a solution to solving the problem. You can do this on your own or with a trusted family member/friend. If you want to expedite the process so you can identify the emotion with the specific pain, I recommend working with a health professional who is trained in Neuro- Emotional Technique. Using this technique in our office, we are able to relieve the pain in minutes by identifying the specific issue and emotion that is associated with your pain.

#3) Learn how to breathe properly to help your body develop more resilience to stress. When people are anxious or stressed, their breathing tends to be more shallow and brief. If you've ever seen anyone have a panic attack, they are hyperventilating and gasping for oxygen to get in their lungs. Counteract that with this simple breathing technique: inhale through your nose for a count of five seconds, hold that breath for five seconds, then exhale through your mouth for a count of five seconds. Do this five times and notice how it puts you in a more relaxed state.

#4) Go for a walk every day. While you're walking, make sure you really swing your arms for an added stress reduction benefit. You can also just get outside in nature and walk barefoot in the park or at the beach.

#5) Do something fun that will include lots of laughter. If you go to the movies, or watch a movie at home, choose a comedy or something that makes you laugh. Laughter is an excellent way of reducing stress. Even the act of laughing out loud without watching anything funny still has a stress relieving benefit to it.

#6) Social interaction with people who support and encourage you is a great way to relieve stress levels. Having a few people over to your house for tea or a casual dinner is a nice way to connect without having to leave your house.

#7) Physical touch in the form of hugging can have wonderful stress relieving benefits. Most people, however, do not hug properly. They hug with their right shoulder over the other person's right shoulder. When you hug someone, hug heart-to-heart with your left shoulder hugging the other person's left shoulder. Try it, it makes a difference.

"I've been seeing Dr. Taylor for 19 years. He has helped me with a lot of different issues ranging from back pain to Lyme disease. Prior to seeing Dr. Taylor, I probably spent over $100,000.00 with different medical clinics and practitioners all around the world. He is the only one who can eliminate my pain, keep my immune system high, figure out and clear my emotional stresses, and keep me riding my horse with no limitations. If he ever moved, I would too. The treatments are that life-changing!" ~Vicki Shinn

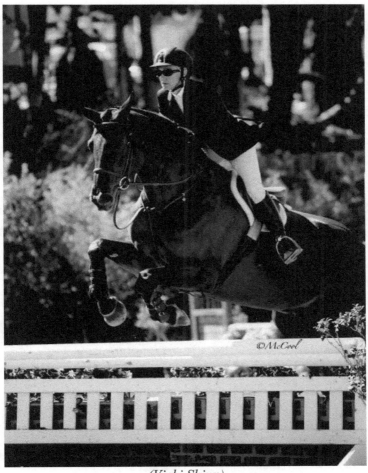

(Vicki Shinn)

Chapter 5

How Water Can Make A Difference In Your Health

"We never know the worth of water until the well is dry."
~Thomas Fuller

"I believe that water is the only drink for a wise man!"
~Henry David Thorough

Water is absolutely essential to staying healthy. In fact, about 65% of your entire body is made up of water. Water helps your body to function properly by lubricating your organs and joints, facilitating digestion, allowing metabolic processes to occur, and eliminating toxins from your body. Water is found in all tissues and organs including the brain, heart, lungs, kidneys, gastrointestinal tract, reproductive organs, eyes, and muscles. Yet, most new patients that step foot in my office are not drinking enough water and present themselves to be in a state of dehydration. Staying hydrated is one of the easiest ways to maintain good health, but many people sabotage their health by not drinking enough water.

How can you tell I'm dehydrated?

When someone comes in my office in pain, 95% of the time they are in a state of dehydration. When you're not drinking enough water, the muscles become more rigid, tight, and tender. If I try to adjust someone when they are in this dehydrated state, nothing happens, and the adjustment bounces back. I tell my patients they have a 'rubber spine.' Also, when patients are dehydrated their brain is stressed and they have a hard time processing, thinking straight, and being 'present.' In addition, when someone has pain in their middle lower back on either side, I suspect that their kidneys are stressed with possible kidney stones, as the kidneys will refer pain to this area. There is a simple test that you can do you to determine if the kidneys are causing the pain. Just place your hand over the area of pain and then giving it a tap with the fist from your other hand. A kidney problem will typically send the patient through the roof if you tap it hard enough.

If you offer up a person in this state a glass of water, they will readily accept it because they are typically thirsty. Your body will typically tell you that it's thirsty when you lose about 2% of your body's water content. Another sign that someone is dehydrated is that they will have dry, cottonmouth with associated bad breath, headaches, and muscle spasms. Stools often become impacted and they present with constipation. They're not going urinate very often, and when they do their urine is dark instead of a pale, light yellow color.

Why am I dehydrated?

Other than the fact that most people do not drink enough water, there are other factors that keep them in the state of dehydration. Every day, your water needs to fluctuate. Warmer days lead to more perspiration which requires more water consumption. Also, perspiration from exercising needs to be replenished so an increase in water needs to take place. Caffeine consumption in the form of coffee, sodas, or tea have a diuretic effect which increases the need for more water. When I tell people they need to drink more water, they often ask, "Do other beverages count such as fruit juice, coffee, or tea?" The answer is 'No.' The only exception is vegetable juice used from greens such as kale, beet tops, spinach, celery, arugula, etc.

The water that comes from these greens is supercharged from the photosynthesis process that comes from the sun, thus giving the body energy and greater hydration.

How much water should I drink per day?

This all depends on your lifestyle and other factors that influence the water percentage in your body.

In general, I typically recommend that my patients drink about half their body weight in fluid ounces. So if a patient weights 150lbs, they should drink approximately 75 ounces of water per day.

If someone is drinking coffee in the morning, I tell them that for every 8 ounces of coffee consumed, drink approximately 32 ounces of water to counter-act the diuretic effect of the coffee they had that morning.

The more dehydrated the individual is, the more they will need to compensate by drinking more water.

Dehydration is typically seen in individuals who lead a very busy lifestyle and consider it an 'inconvenience' to always 'have to be going to the bathroom' because they drink too much water.

My patients who are teachers are famous for not drinking enough water because they cannot leave their classroom seven times a day to excuse themselves.

Children are also prone to be dehydrated because they simply do not drink enough water.

People who eat a lot of starches in the form of breads, pastas, cookies, and processed food, are often dehydrated as this food absorbs much water in the large intestine.

Those who are older are often dehydrated as their thirst mechanism becomes weaker with age. For this reason, the elderly need to make more of a concerted effort to drink water, especially if they are consuming prescription medications that have a tendency to dehydrate them even more.

Ultimately, your body will let you know how much water to drink each day. When the water content in your body drops about 2%, your thirst mechanism will activate. Immediately drink water when you sense your need for it and don't put off or ignore what your body is trying to tell you.

Is it possible to drink too much water?

Your body is a balance of electrolytes...Sodium, Potassium, Magnesium, Phosphate, Chlorine, and Calcium are just a few. Drinking too much water for your body to handle can cause an imbalance in your sodium potassium levels and cause a condition called Hyponatremia. Headaches, confusion, fatigue, lack of energy, irritability, and muscle spasms are some of the symptoms of this condition. Your kidneys, when they are functioning properly, can process the water you are drinking at a decent rate. However, if your kidneys are not functioning properly and you drink too much water, too quickly, this can lead to water intoxication and cause Hyponatremia. To be on the safe side, it is recommended to drink less than 20 ounces of water per hour so your kidneys have time to excrete and process the water you consume.

In Summary:

In summary, drinking enough water each day is essential to good health. It is one of the simplest things you can do to stay healthy and yet many people fail to do so. In general, your body will tell you how much water you should drink per day by following your thirst mechanism. When you're thirsty, drink water. You know you're not getting enough water if your urine is a dark yellow and you're not urinating much during the day. You should be urinating consistently throughout the day. Drinking too much water, too quickly, can create an electrolyte imbalance, particularly a condition called Hyponatremia. Ideally, drink less than 20 ounces of water per hour so your kidneys have time to process the water.

"Over the years I've referred many patients to Dr. Taylor, of whom only have great things to say about him. Dr. Taylor is not only compassionate with these patients, but provides treatments that makes them want to come back and continue care with him as he improves their lifestyle."

Dr. Peter S. Borden, M.D.
Orthopedic Surgeon
Orthopedic Sports Medicine, Shoulder and Knee Specialist.
Owner of Sports and Spine Orthopedic Clinic

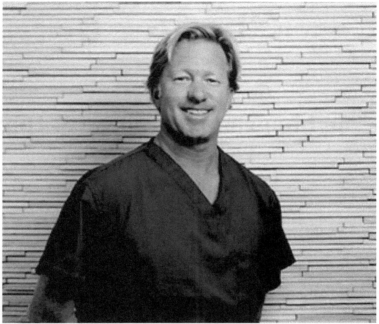

(Dr. Peter S. Borden, M.D.)

Chapter 6

The Importance Of Sleep & How To Improve It

"You're not healthy, unless your sleep is healthy."
~ Dr. William Dement, father of sleep medicine

"A good laugh and a long sleep
are the best cures in the doctor's book."
~ Irish Proverb

Getting a good night's rest on a regular basis is essential to experiencing excellent health. There have been many studies demonstrating that sleep deprivation has been linked to heart disease, diabetes, a weakened immune system and even an increased risk for cancer. Not getting enough sleep has also been associated with a poor mental and emotional state of mind which leads to poor decision-making, decreased creativity, and more mistakes on the job.

Proper rest is essential as your body detoxifies through the night and physiologically repairs itself. Failure to get adequate sleep puts your body and mind in a more vulnerable state, making you more susceptible to health problems and disease. Over the past 25 years, I've had patients come in who did not get much sleep the night before and it was almost like they were drunk, extra edgy, in more pain, and more tense.

A well-rested individual displays the opposite. Sound mind, more at ease, less pain, and more relaxed.

So how much rest is really needed per night?

On average, my patients seem to do well with 7 to 8 hours of sleep per night. The younger my patient is, of course, the more rest they are going to need. Newborns, infants, and toddlers need 10-13 hours of sleep per night, while young children and teenagers typically need 9 to 12 hours of sleep per night. The older you get, typically the less sleep you need. Too much sleep also can work against you when you are older and throw off your circadian rhythms, having similar detrimental effects as sleep deprivation. Just because

8 hours of sleep is good for you, it doesn't mean that 10 or 12 hours is even better.

What if I can't sleep at night?

If you are not sleeping well at night, you need to find the cause of why you're not sleeping and work towards getting that corrected. Failure to sleep is often associated with hormonal imbalances including high cortisol production released by the adrenal glands. Your adrenal glands respond to stress, so the more stressed you are, the greater chances you have of sleeping less. Your pineal gland in your brain also may not be producing enough melatonin to help you sleep. Not getting enough sunlight during the day and exposing yourself to artificial lights during the night can affect your melatonin production, therefore affecting your sleep as well as your body's ability to fight cancer. Consuming caffeinated beverages and eating a diet high in sugar and carbohydrates can definitely affect the quality of your sleep. The bottom line is that no matter what health condition you are struggling with at this time, if you're not sleeping well, it will only make your problem worse.

What can I do to improve the quality of my sleep?

There are a number of things that you can do to improve the quality of your sleep.

1) Make sure to start the day right by getting adequate sunlight. The brighter the sunlight, the greater the stimulation to the pineal gland to secrete melatonin.

2) Exercise by taking a walk first thing in the morning, at noon, and in the evening to reduce stress and expose your eyes to the sunlight at different times of the day.

3) Improve your diet by decreasing sugar and carbohydrate consumption, as well as any foods you may be sensitive to such as gluten and dairy.

4) Eliminate caffeinated beverages such as coffee and sodas as well as food with caffeine such as chocolate in the afternoon. Some people may have their sleep affected even by drinking caffeine in the morning. If this is the case with you, eliminate it all together.

5) Work towards eliminating the mental and emotional stressors in your life that increase stress levels by talking them out with a trusted family member, friend, or other confidant.

6) Develop an evening routine that helps you get in a pattern for sleep: DON'T watch TV or be on your

phone/computer right before bed, or eat right before going to bed. DO wind down with a hot shower, and/or read before bed, which is a very helpful aid in falling asleep.

7) Make sure the temperature in your room is not too hot, but a little on the cooler side -approximately in the mid 60's for optimal sleep.

8) Try to go to bed and wake up at the same time to establish a routine that will help your body get in a pattern for sleep.

9) Make sure it is completely dark in your room, as light can pass through the eyelid and disrupt the pineal gland in producing melatonin at night. Make sure no light from any electronic device is on in your room as well as any light coming in through the window. If you have a skylight in the ceiling or cannot make the room completely dark, invest in a high quality blackout mask.

10) Do not have any electronic devices near your head such as your clock radio, cell phone with charger plugged into the wall, or even sleep with your head near a light switch or outlet. Some people are very sensitive to EMF's (Electromagnetic Frequency) and the slightest stimulation can affect their sleep.

11) Do not use any electric heating blankets in the winter.

12) Go to sleep when you start feeling tired. Don't fight it, but listen to your body when it is telling you to go to sleep. For example, if you are feeling tired at 9:00PM, go to bed at that time. If you stay up past that time, you may lose that sleepiness and your second wind kicks in, resulting in you not feeling tired again till midnight or even later.

13) Don't drink anything a few hours before going to bed to avoid getting up in the middle of the night to use the bathroom. Failure to get into a deep sleep because you have to get up a few times in the night greatly affects the quality of your sleep.

14) Make it a point to get up earlier, which typically has an effect of making you go to bed earlier. This goes back to your body working in harmony with circadian rhythms. Go to bed when the sun goes down and wake up when the sun arises. Typically, the later you get up in the morning, the easier it is to stay up later at night. The earlier you go to bed, the greater rest your body gets as more efficient repair occurs before midnight. Also, your cortisol levels typically are at their lowest around 10PM.

15) Try sleeping on your right side, as it is easier on the body. You will see that it is typically easier to breathe with your heart on top, above the liver, rather than the other way around.

I do NOT recommend any Fitbit device, as the negative electromagnetic energy that emits from these are incredibly strong. The negative energy emitted from these devices are not worth the information you receive from them, in exchange for putting your health in jeopardy. I have had too many patients come in who have tested so weak with these devices and had no idea it was making them weaker, putting their health at risk.

What if I tried all those suggestions and still can't get to sleep?

Sometimes, people try all of the suggestions above and still have a problem going to sleep. If this is the case, seeking out professional help may be needed to help you overcome the insomnia. Initially, you may want to have your nervous system balanced with chiropractic care and therapeutic massage to release adhesive scar tissue that is keeping your body in a state of tension and stress. By doing this, it can have a great effect on relieving your adrenal glands and help you get to sleep.

What should I do if chiropractic care and therapeutic massage do not help me overcome the insomnia?

If you still have problems going to sleep after getting under chiropractic care, you may have to go to the next level and treat the brain directly with Neuro-Integrative Therapy. Neuro- Integrative Therapy is a form of neurofeedback using photonics that corrects irregular brain waves and modifies timing patterns in the brain. Sometimes, people's Delta brain waves get out of rhythm with their Alpha, Beta, and Theta brain waves, making it impossible for them to go to sleep. This retraining occurs over multiple Neuro-Integrative Therapy sessions and the brain is retrained into normal patterns. The result is an improvement in brain regulation, which often leads to wonderful, sound, and deep sleep.

This technology has over 40 years of clinical research and studies to demonstrate its effectiveness. And the best part about it is that it is non-invasive, uses no drugs, and often makes permanent changes in the brain. The results I have seen at our clinic using this technology has been nothing short of amazing!

"When I first started seeing Dr. Taylor, I could barely walk because of my left knee pain. I used to come to work using a cane to get there, then I would hide my cane so others would not see me using it. After receiving treatments with Dr. Taylor's techniques and different technology, my knee pain eventually went away. I also lost all the achy joints and stiff muscles in my hips, lower back and shoulders. Dr. Taylor also put me on his weight loss program and since I started care with him, I've lost 65lbs and I continue to lose the weight. Before seeing Dr. Taylor, I also had problems sleeping all my life and would wake up every few hours, never being able to sleep through the night. Over the last 8 years, my sleep has gotten worse. I started using his new brain enhancement technology and after the first treatment, I slept a whole 5 hours straight. I now am able to sleep 8 hours/night and I've never had such deep sleep in all my life. Since I'm getting more sleep, my brain works better, my mood has been enhanced, I have more energy, and overall, I feel like a whole new person."

~Dr. Laura Den Blaker, D.C.

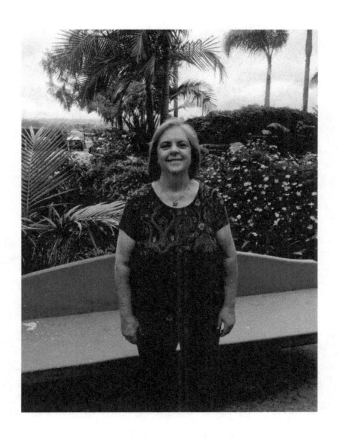

(Dr. Laura Den Blaker, D.C.)

CHAPTER 7

Exercise:
Work Smarter, Not Harder

*"It is a shame for a man to grow old
without seeing the beauty and strength
of which his body is capable."*
~Socrates

*"Those who think they have no time for exercise
will sooner or later have to find time for illness."*
~Edward Stanley

In this chapter, I would like to address two types of exercises I recommend for my patients. The first type of exercise has to do with pain relief, and the second type of exercise has to do with longevity. Over the past 25 years of practice, by far the most common question I hear from my patients is, "What exercises can I do to get better faster?" I tell them this depends on what muscle is causing the problem and what muscle needs to be addressed.

When I first started out in practice I would give patients a generic handout of common exercises anyone can do for the low back, neck, shoulder, or other area of complaint. What I discovered was that these exercises were helpful for some patients, but for other patients it made them worse. The best exercises are going to be specific for what each individual patient's body presents. I suppose this is why patients are constantly asking, "What type of exercises can I do?" They've been burned before by doing an exercise that was recommended by a professional, but it turned out hurting them more than helping them.

There are a myriad of exercises you can do for each condition you may be dealing with; however, in this chapter I'd like to share with you the most common and effective exercises that I found to help patients get better. The first thing you need to understand is that your body must be properly aligned. If it's out of alignment and you have postural distortions and imbalances you'll experience pain. So the key is to find the right exercises to get your body back in balance.

In a previous chapter I had you look in the mirror to see if you have any structural imbalances. Notice if your head is tilted to the right or the left. Is it rotated to the left or the right? Is it leaning forward or sitting backwards on your shoulders? Next you'll want to look at your shoulders again. Is one higher than the other? Is one rotated more on one side?

Next, look at your hips. Place your hands at the top of your waist and feel the bones of your hip underneath your hands. Now, while looking in the mirror is one hand higher than the other? Go down and look at your knees. They should be pointing at a 10° angle laterally. Are they symmetrical? Is one knee rotated outward or inward more than the other? Lastly, look at your feet. Your feet are the foundation of your spine. Is one foot laterally rotated more than the other? Are your feet flat? Can you fit your fingers underneath the middle of your arch?

After looking at your body this way, what do you observe? If there are quite a few postural distortions, you'll be wearing out your joints quicker than you should, and you'll be heading down the road to pain.

These postural distortions will also give you a clue on what you're doing repetitively during the day that may be contributing to your imbalances. For example, I have a patient who is a dental hygienist and is constantly twisting her body to the left to work on her patients' teeth. Her postural distortions demonstrate what she's doing all day long for eight hours, especially on the days she sees eight patients a day, back to back. If she works three days a week and has a packed schedule like this, 24 hours a week she's bent over and stooped in this position.

Do you think this influences her posture? Do you think this can create adhesions and imbalances that lead to pain? The answer of course is, 'Yes!' So, the key exercises she should be doing are the ones that will counteract these habitual repetitive patterns. She can do upper body trunk twists periodically throughout the day, especially on the days when she's working as a hygienist. And she can do this in between patients. It would probably take 30 seconds to perform a set of 20 repetitions.

Finding the appropriate exercise for your condition is a simple concept that once you understand it can make a profound impact on your alignment. As you can see the exercise routine needs to be customized based upon your postural imbalances and distortions. If your head is rotated to the left, your exercises should be to rotate your head to the right. If your right shoulder is internally rotated, your exercises should be to externally rotate that shoulder.

Now, there's a proper way to do the exercises which I don't have space to show you in this book. And I don't want to overload you with 500 different exercises to perform. But I would like to give you a few examples which I've found to be extremely helpful for the most common conditions and painful areas in the body that I see in my practice. In addition, even if you don't have pain in these areas, these are good exercises to maintain good posture and can be used to prevent negative conditions.

Let's start from the top:

NECK: I've discovered that most people with neck pain are dealing with problems in the muscles of the lateral neck (scalenes and sternocleidomastoid), as well as muscles in the front of the chest (pectoralis major and minor). The first stretch I would do is a pec stretch using a door frame as your anchor. Hold your arm at 90° in place on a door frame. Lean forward and gently stretch this muscle. Hold for a count of 20 seconds.

The next exercise I would do for the neck would be a chin retraction. Look straight ahead. Bring your chin back as far as you can while keeping the chin parallel to the floor. In other words, don't tilt your head back or forward, but keep it level.

SHOULDERS: Most people with shoulder problems are stuck in internal rotation. So the best exercise for shoulders is to facilitate external rotation. A great exercise is to stretch out both arms to your side and parallel with the floor with thumbs pointing behind you. Slowly do arm circles in small slows circles for 30 seconds. This can be performed a few times per day.

HIPS: Most people's hips are very tight and are causing stress and strain on the low back, knees, and even neck/shoulders. An easy stretch to keep the hips loose is a standing wall stretch.

If you're trying to stretch out your right hip, stand parallel to the wall and place your right foot approximately 2 feet away from the wall. Cross your left foot over your right foot, then place your right hand/forearm on the wall. Lean your hips toward the wall and hold in this position for 20 seconds. Do the same for the opposite hip.

LOWER BACK: When someone comes in with lower back pain, I've discovered that the area of complaint is rarely the muscle that needs to be stretched or exercised. Lower back pain typically comes from these four muscles: **#1** the psoas major (hip flexors); **#2** the lower rectus abdominis (lower stomach muscles); **#3** the gluteus maximus (rear end); **#4** the quadriceps (thighs). Other common muscles are the piriformis and gluteus medius.

The number one stretch I've found helpful for low back pain is the psoas stretch. This can be performed on a bench, bed, or floor. If performing it on the floor, place one knee on the floor and the other foot stretched out before you. Lean forward until you feel a gentle stretch of the psoas muscle (the hip flexor found where your thigh connects to your waist). Hold for 20 seconds. Perform this stretch three times per day.

The next stretch I like is stretching the glutes with an L stretch. Place your leg in an L-shaped pattern on the floor and lean forward. Hold for 20 seconds. Perform this three times per day.

KNEES: Adhesions found in the quadriceps muscles can refer pain and tightness to the knees. It is important to keep these muscles stretched out. A very simple and common stretch for the knee is a standing quadriceps stretch. If you want to stretch out the right knee, stand on your left leg, bend your right knee, and grab your right foot with your right hand to stretch out that quad. Hold for 20 seconds and repeat with the other leg.

These are a few of the more common stretches I recommend to alleviate pain and to prevent conditions from occurring. Once a patient is out of pain, the next question is, "What's the best way for me to exercise to maintain overall good health and longevity?"

Everyone knows it's almost impossible to stay healthy without doing some type of exercise. Exercise keeps you young, slows down the aging process, keeps you fit, and stimulates growth hormone which is your body's most important anti-aging hormone.

Exercising on a regular basis increases longevity and improves the quality of your life, yet many do not exercise as much as they should or do not know the best and most efficient way to exercise.

I started seriously exercising when I entered high school. I played football and ran track so my main source of exercise was weightlifting and cardiovascular work. This carried on in my college years and young adult life.

Like every young man, I lifted weights for the purpose of gaining muscle size and not for the purpose of being healthy. I figured if I had a strong looking physique, then I would naturally be healthy on the inside.

The latest research demonstrates the opposite. Larger muscles developed by lifting heavy weights have shown that the tensile strength of those fibers diminish with aging and the effects of heavy lifting do not benefit you when you are older.

I never understood this until I started doing the research on exercise, muscle fibers, and longevity.

I'm at a different stage in my life where my main focus is to increase my health and longevity. I'm assuming that this is also the goal of most of you reading this book.

What type of exercise should I do increase my longevity and overall health?

When it comes to exercise, don't make the same mistake I did for years by jogging for cardiovascular health and lifting weights for bodybuilding purposes.

In our fast and busy lifestyle, who has time to spend three hours jogging per week and two hours in the gym three times a week?

If you are really pressed for time and happen to be the type who does not exercise because you're too busy, there are no more excuses as you can actually effectively exercise in as little as ONE HOUR per week if you do it right.

How can you effectively exercise and maintain good health by only exercising ONE HOUR per week you ask?

The answer is you have to work smarter, not harder.

All the latest research demonstrates that high intensity interval training yields the greatest results for overall health.

What is high intensity interval training?

High-intensity interval training is working your body on an anaerobic level by doing a high intensity, short burst of exercise for 20 to 30 seconds followed by 90 seconds of rest and recovery. It is recommended to warm up for about 5 minutes prior to starting this process. If you combine the warm-up and repeat this process seven times, you've just completed an incredible workout routine in about 20 minutes.

Here's an example workout session for high intensity interval training:

1. Perform a 5 minute warm-up such as walking, treadmill, cycling, anything to get the blood and circulation going.
2. Choose an exercise and go as intense and fast as you can for 30 seconds. How do you know that you have reached the right intensity? You will be feeling out of breath towards the end of the exercise and feel a

burn in the muscles you are using. If you check your pulse, it should be at your maximum heart rate :
(220 – Age = MHR).

3. Rest & Recover for 90 seconds
4. Repeat the same procedure of exercise and recovery for a total of 7 times.

When you're first starting out, you may not be able to go a full 7 times. You may have to start out by doing 2 to 3 cycles and work your way up to 7 cycles. Be careful to not overdo it and potentially injure yourself by straining a muscle. This is why it is important to warm-up first and listen to your body. Overdoing it will only set you back and prevent you from reaching your goals.

High intensity interval training should only be performed every other day, as your body needs to rest and heal for at least 48 hours after the exercise. Don't think that just because a little bit is good for me a lot is going to be even better. It doesn't work that way. Proper rest and recovery is essential.

In regards to the exercise you use, if you have a stationary bike or belong to a fitness facility, you can use a stair stepper, elliptical machine, upper body ergometer, or any of the equipment that you can do a very fast-paced exercise on without injuring yourself.

If you do not have exercise equipment, you can perform these types of exercises by doing a very fast brisk walk, jumping jacks, running in place, or even sprinting. You must be very careful to be properly warmed-up and not injure and/or over-exert yourself by trying to do too much when your body is not ready for it.

It is important to note that after doing an intense exercise such as this, your body will be recovering for the next few hours. You're going to want to eat, and it is very imperative that you stay away from gluten, carbohydrates, and sugars, including fruit juices. A trip to the local juice store after performing high intensity interval training exercise will undo all the hard work you just performed. Gluten, carbohydrates, and sugars will prevent the production of human growth hormone and all the hard work you just did to stimulate human growth hormone, which is your number one antiaging hormone, which will go out the window when you eat the wrong food. This is why it is said that the best workout routine cannot outdo a bad diet.

It is important that you mix up the exercises and get a variety of different types of routines so your body receives the maximum benefit from a variety of different stresses placed upon it. Performing the identical daily exercise routine does not challenge the body in the same way that a variety of exercises can achieve.

There are **three types of muscle fibers** that should be utilized for an overall strengthening of the body:

1. **Slow Twitch Red Muscle Fibers** are activated with aerobic, endurance type exercises. These fibers are filled with plenty of capillaries and mitochondria, and contain a lot of oxygen.

2. **Fast Twitch Red Muscle Fibers**, which are also activated with aerobic and strength training type exercises, also have a lot of capillaries and mitochondria but are much faster than the slow twitch muscle fibers. Power training, or weight training-burst types of exercises, will activate the fast twitch muscle fibers.

3. **Extremely Fast Twitch White Muscle Fibers** are activated with anaerobic short bursts of exercises. These fibers do not contain much blood supply and have less mitochondria to utilize so they burn out faster. High Interval Intense Training activate these fibers.

When you actively incorporate all three types of muscle fibers and utilize both aerobic and anaerobic training, you provide a well-rounded balance and strength to the body, keeping it at top performance.

What is the smartest way to perform strength training and muscular development?

High intensity strength training, which is different from regular strength training, in that you are trying to intentionally maximize the use of the muscle by lifting the weight very slowly so that the muscle fatigues very profoundly and quickly at the same time. This creates a metabolic effect that has many benefits to the body, such as decreasing body fat, lowering your risk for diabetes, improving your immune system, and even fighting against cancer.

High intensity strength training (using weights, machines, or a chin up bar at a gradual & slow pace) is also different from high intensity interval training (using a stationary bike, cardiovascular machine, sprinting, etc. with short bursts of rapid movement). High intensity strength training using a gradual and slow pace is safer than high intensity interval training with a quick and ballistic approach.

Here's an example workout session for high intensity strength training using a chin-up bar & dumbbells:

. 1. Stand on a chair, under a chin up bar. Grab the bar with your palms facing towards you in the supinated position. Slowly do a pull up at a very slow pace, 10 seconds to come up. Then lower yourself slowly, 10 seconds to go down. Repeat the process and as your muscles start to fatigue assist yourself up by using the chair. When you first start, start very slowly where it takes three seconds to barely come up and down. With each rep, your muscles should fatigue to the point where you start to feel an intense burning. The goal is to have a deep level of fatigue where the stimulus of the exercise creates the positive metabolic response. The amount of reps or the time spent doing the exercise is not as important as achieving the goal of having a deep level of fatigue. Unlike the high intensity interval training, this is not a 30 second set with a 90 second rest.

2. Grab two dumbbells, sit on a bench, and slowly start to push up, performing a military press. This should take about 10 seconds to accomplish. Slowly, bring the dumbbells down. Repeat the process until you reach the deep level of fatigue which typically should be at least a

minimum of 4 reps. You may have to lower the weight if you are doing less than 4 reps.

3. Grab a gym ball and place it behind your back with your knees and hips flexed at 90° while holding a dumbbell. You're in a sitting position without a chair beneath you and statically hold this position for as long as you can. Start to perform very slow deep knee bends and push back up until you can no longer do this.

4. Grab your two dumbbells and begin performing a chest press starting very slowly to push them up but do not let the dumbbells hit each other, make sure to keep the space between them about 8 inches wide. Slowly return the dumbbells back down but do not let them rest by bringing them all the way back. Repeat the process to fatigue.

5. Grab one dumbbell, hold the dumbbell between both hands and slowly start to lower the dumbbell where it goes beyond your head, then bring the dumbbell back where it is over your chest again. Repeat the process to fatigue.

You can modify this routine in the gym with machines. You're basically trying to stress all the major muscles of the body by doing a vertical pulling motion - a chin-up or pulldown, a vertical pushing motion - a military press, a squat or leg press, a horizontal pushing motion – a chest press, and a horizontal pulling motion – a row. The first inch of the movement should take about three seconds, after the body starts to fatigue a little you can push as hard as you can because you will not be able to push at a fast rate. Try to keep the same form and high level of effort throughout the exercises.

High intensity strength training only needs to be performed once a week and the whole routine should take less than 14 minutes, as each set will most likely be less than 2 minutes. Remember, the intent of the exercises is to perform it the hardest way possible so the muscles are continuously loaded and you achieve a rapid and deep level of fatigue.

In addition to the high intensity interval training and high intensity strength training, I would also advise you to perform an aerobic exercise such as walking, brisk walking, jogging, and exercise cardio machines to help develop the slow twitch red muscle fibers and increase oxygen to the body, improving stamina and strengthening the immune system.

It is also a good idea to strengthen your core muscles in your mid-section, such as the muscles of the lower back, hips, and abdomen, and stretch out your chronically shortened muscles caused by the activities of daily living, such as the hip flexors and quads. This will help prevent injury to the back and reduce pain caused by shortened muscles with adhesive scar tissue.

Now, although it is important to incorporate all these exercises, understand that when you activate the fast twitch red muscle fibers and very fast twitch white muscle fibers when using the high intensity training, you have the potential to release human growth hormone which is your primary antiaging hormone. By performing these exercises you will slow down the aging process, decrease body fat, increase mental capacity, increase energy levels, firm up skin tonality, and basically look and feel younger.

An important caveat to mention is that when you do this type of exercise, it should be on an empty stomach while intermittently fasting. When you have food in your stomach while you're working out it will prevent your cells from repairing and rebuilding themselves which defeats the purpose of the work out. Instead of your body using fat for fuel, it will use glucose or sugars, which in turn will give you a craving for sugar after your workout.

Having sugar in your system will also prevent human growth hormone from being released and you lose the benefits of your high-intensity training workout.

In summary: If you're doing exercises to get out of pain, first look in the mirror and see where your postural distortions are located. Then proceed to perform an exercise that will provide the opposite effect of your postural distortion. When you are done with this exercise, you should see an improvement and change in your posture. If you're doing exercises for longevity, you don't need to spend a lot of time exercising in order to receive the benefits of keeping your body young, healthy, and pain free. High-intensity training in the form of high intensity interval training and high intensity strength training can be done in as little as one hour per week. Two-20 minute sessions of high intensity interval training a week plus one-14 minute session of high-intensity strength training is all you need to stimulate human growth hormone which is your primary antiaging hormone. Human growth hormone helps your body to burn fat, improve skin tonality, increase energy levels, and keeps you looking and feeling young. The effects of this training can be ruined, however, by eating gluten, carbohydrates, or sugar after your workout. It is best to have an easily digestible, high-quality protein source after working out to help your muscles repair, such as Solutions4 whey protein shakes that have casein and lactose removed. Regular protein such as beef, chicken, and fish takes too long to assimilate after a workout and you do not receive the benefit of replenishing your broken down protein. Remember that exercise produces a catabolic effect and failure to have protein in the hours after an acute workout can potentially waste and damage your muscles, so do not neglect this important component of your workout routine.

"I have an ongoing knee issue that I've had for many years. In 1969, I was a walk on at the University of Oklahoma and injured my knee my freshman year of playing football. It was a serious injury. As I got older, I would try to jog to stay in shape, but the pain just became too much. If I over exerted it, it would swell up and I would be off my feet for a few days in pain. Dr. Taylor treated my knee and it made a remarkable difference. The next morning when I woke up I had to think to myself for a moment and remind myself which knee was my bad knee. That's how much satisfaction and

relief I received. I feel no pain going downstairs. I've had no swelling on the knee. I can now kneel on my knee without pain. I was skeptical at first, but seeing is believing. My pain is virtually gone. I am able to resume many of my normal activities."

~Dennis Bales, Spin Instructor & Creative Innovator of 'Spinning to the Hits'

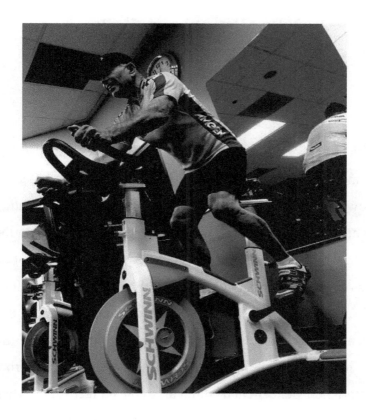

(Dennis Bales)

Chapter 8

Sitting? Get Out Of That Chair!

"There is a point in every contest
when sitting on the sidelines is not an option."
~Dean Smith

In the last chapter, much time was devoted to discuss the life-changing benefits that proper exercise can do for your health. However, all the hard work you put into exercise and eating right can be destroyed by simply sitting too much during the day. Most people have no idea that too much sitting is often the root cause of many chronic health problems, as millions of Americans unknowingly suffer the consequences of this silent but deadly activity. Sitting has become a part of life we just don't think about and it is slowly robbing us from experiencing excellent health. Part of the danger is that when a person gets there half hour or hour of exercise in that morning, they think that they don't have to do any other physical activity until their next workout routine. They don't realize that a 45 minute exercise routine will not offset eight hours or more of sitting in a chair.

Why shouldn't I sit if I have a back problem?

First of all, sitting can have detrimental effects to the spine as it reverses the lordotic curve in your lumbar and cervical spine which puts undue stress on the discs, ligaments, tendons, and muscles associated with the spine. This can lead to pain, headaches, and overall poor health function. Sitting for long periods of time also puts pressure, stresses, and tensions on the body which can cause pain and dysfunction. What makes it worse and accentuates the problem is, the more you weigh and the heavier you are, the more pressure, pain, and damage you will experience in the lower back. Additionally, the less cushion and give the chair has to offer, the more problems you will experience as well. These facts are based on Newton's Third Law of Motion, which states that every action has an equal and opposite reaction. If you don't believe me, try this. Sit on a hard chair. Notice the pressure and tension you feel in the middle of your lower back. Now shift your weight to your left gluteus maximus. Notice how the tension translated from the middle lower back to the left side of the lower back. Now place a soft, spongy pad underneath your bottom and see how the tension lessens when you sit. The softer the surface is that you sit on, the less pressure you should feel in your back. The only problem with this is that you have to take into consideration the importance of proper posture. Sitting on a chair that is too soft, without structural support, will contribute to poor posture. Poor posture will add new stresses to the spine and create problems for you. For example, sit in a chair and instead of sitting upright, (by the way, the proper posture for sitting is to sit up tall as if you are trying to see over a fence, but with your eyes level) slouch in your seat with poor posture and notice the new tensions that occur in your lower back as a result of slouching. The longer you sit, the more those tensions translate up from the lower back to the mid back to the neck and beyond, yes, even to the bones and tissues associated with the cranium. By the way, these principles also apply for standing, walking, exercise routines, etc. This is why it is important to be posturally aware of what is going on with your body at all times. Failure to pay attention and be aware of the stresses you feel in your body, inevitably leads to problems.

How is sitting associated with other health problems?

Sitting puts your body and nervous system in a state of rest, shutting down molecular activity and affecting all tissues at a cellular level. When this happens, it can affect your endocrine system as well as other organs and systems of the body. Prolonged sitting has been associated with pain, metabolic syndrome, high blood pressure, poor circulation, and an increase in free radical production, which is associated with cancer.

Studies have shown that after prolonged sitting, the body goes in a state of rest. However, when a person stands up after being seated, muscular and cellular systems that regulate blood sugar and cholesterol are activated and mediated through insulin.

This is why walking and exercise is recommended by health practitioners to help regulate blood sugars.

Walking helps to assimilate your nutrition into the cells and help the body to function optimally.

Sitting does the opposite as all your cellular mechanisms get switched off and blood sugar and cholesterol levels rise with sitting. Increase that to prolonged sitting for 12 hours per day, 5 to 6 days per week, for years and even decades, you start to develop a host of metabolic and other health problems. Researchers say that the ratio for sitting and premature death is 2:1. In other words, for every hour a person sits, you can shave two hours off that person's life. There is even an interesting study found that smokers were healthier than non-smokers because the smokers were forced to get off their chairs and walk to a designated area where they could smoke. The study concluded that taking more breaks and being more physically active, such as getting up from a chair to take a break, produced positive health benefits even in people who were smokers over those who were more sedentary and non-smokers. A recent study published in the British Medical Journal discovered that one of the greatest tests/indicators for morbidity and longevity involves how many times within the span of a minute, you are able to stand up and sit back down in a chair. Another study shows that your ability to get off the floor from seated position is a good predictor for early mortality. If you have to use both hands and knees or something to help you get off the floor, it's not a good sign of health.

So what should be done to solve the problem of too much sitting?

The average American office worker sits for approximately 13 hours a day. What should you do if you are in this situation? You have to get up and move more. At a bare minimum, you should set the timer on your phone to go off every 25 minutes so you can get up and perform a few simple exercises, such as jumping jacks, squats, toe touchers, or any other type of exercise that helps get the circulation going. Another option is to purchase a Swiss gym ball and use that as your chair. If you were to do this, make sure to get a Swiss gym ball that is a little taller than the one you exercise on so that you can let out some of the air, making it more comfortable, where your legs and hips are at a 90° angle. Make sure your gym ball is an anti-burst Dura Pro ball, so that just in case it pops you don't injure yourself. This ball will deflate slowly rather than suddenly if damage is done to it. Ideally, you want to sit as little as possible during the day, so if neither of these options will work for you the best option is to get a standup desk and not sit at all. Standup desks range from a few hundred dollars to over one thousand dollars depending on your needs. If you cannot afford for a standup desk at this time, you can always create your own by putting your computer on an upside down box or clear plastic bin.

Won't I create another problem if I'm standing on my feet all day?

It is true that prolonged standing can also cause back and joint pain along with other problems, so make sure you have a padded surface to stand on to take the pressure off your joints. Make sure that you are constantly shifting your weight appropriately so that you're not standing in one place for too long in the same spot at one time. It will benefit you to be barefoot at your standup desk, however, if your work does not allow you to do this, make sure you're not wearing high heels or poor quality shoes that are going to compromise your joints and spine. On a side note, standing will activate your brain and nervous system, allowing you to be more productive and providing better brain function. It will also help your body to burn and utilize fat more efficiently, naturally leading to less body fat and weight loss.

When you first start to replace sitting with standing, your body will not be used to it. You need to break in this new, positive habit slowly and not overdo it. Your back, joints, and tissues will be deconditioned and unable to withstand the new forces you will place on it by standing.

You may want to start out by standing for 15 minutes a day and increase that each day by 10 minutes until you reach your desired target. If there are any areas that are sore or tight at the end of the day, you can use a tennis ball to work out some of the soreness and follow it up immediately with a stretch to that muscle.

To ease the transition from sitting to standing you can immediately start to incorporate exercises that will take the pressure off your low back while standing. One simple exercise to do is marching in place while bringing the knees up so that your hips and knees are at a 90° angle. You can march up and down for one minute at a time and then rest.

Another simple exercise is to keep your leg straight and move it behind you, extending the hip. Squeeze your gluteus maximus when you do this activity and it will help firm and tone your buttocks as well. Perform this for one minute at a time and then rest.

You can also laterally kick out your leg, performing an abduction of the hip. This is a great exercise to reduce the tension developed in the hips and will often give you a good burn while doing them since they are often so deconditioned.

What exercises can I do while sitting?

Standing is always the preferable option, however, if you have to sit, do not sit in one position and slouch for more than 15 minutes at a time. Performing exercises while sitting can help you take some pressure off of the disc, ligaments, and connective tissue of the lower back.

Ideally, sitting on a Swiss gym ball is always optimal when performing exercises while sitting. However, if you are unable to use a Swiss gym ball, you can still perform these exercises while sitting in a chair. Just like the standing exercises you can do a seated march, lifting your leg up one at a time while sitting. Perform this for 1 minute and rest. Next, you can tilt your pelvis forward and backward while keeping an upright posture. Picture your pelvis being a fishbowl and when you are doing a forward tilt, you are spilling the water out of the bowl onto your lap. When you are doing a backward tilt, imagine the water spilling behind your seat. Do this exercise for 30 seconds at a time and perform it throughout the day. The next exercise is a side to side tilt where you are lifting up your pelvis side to side. Imagine that a string is tied to each crest of your hip and someone is alternately lifting up each string as if you are a puppet. Perform this activity for 30 seconds at a time and perform it throughout the day. The next exercise is a pelvic circle where you are moving your pelvis in a circular motion. Imagine you are stirring a pot of soup using your hips. Rotate your hips in a clockwise motion 10 times, followed by a counter-clockwise motion 10 times. Perform this activity throughout the day. Lastly, you can make figure-eight's with your pelvis and do this for 30 seconds at a time and perform it throughout the day.

In summary: Sitting is one of the most subtle and silent forms of slowly degenerating your health and decreasing the years of your life. You must be aware of its damaging effects and make every effort to not sit for more than three hours a day. Turn your workstation into a standing desk and remember that you do not have to invest in expensive furniture to accomplish this. A plastic bin from the store can accomplish this or even a cardboard box. Whether you're sitting or standing, be mindful of the pressures that are exerted on your body and work towards making shifts through exercise and body positions to alleviate these tensions. If you follow this piece of advice alone it can make great strides in your overall health.

"Dr. Taylor has an innate, sixth sense and he has the ability to center me physically and emotionally every time I come to

see him. Whenever I have a pain, he is able to zero in on the problem and take care of it for me. I have referred a number of patients to his office and they are happy as well, as he is able to find the root cause of their pain too. I've suffered permanent neck damage as a result of a car accident and I was injured at another chiropractic office, but Dr. Taylor has never hurt my neck in all the years I have seen him and I've been coming to him since 1998. Thank you Dr. Taylor!"
~Jodi Wiggins, Artist

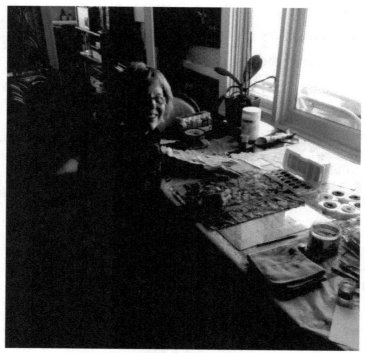

(Jodi Wiggins)

Chapter 9

Sunlight: Vitamin D Is Free - If You Want To Live A Long Life It Is Key!

"The Sun, with all those planets revolving around it, and dependent upon it, can still ripen a bunch of grapes as if it had nothing else in the universe to do."

~Galileo, Astronomer

One of the simplest and most overlooked ways to get healthy is to make sure you get adequate Vitamin D by exposing yourself to sunlight. Next to a healthy diet, exercise, hydration, and sleep, getting adequate Vitamin D in sunshine is one of the most important things you can do for your health.

Why is vitamin D so important?

Vitamin D3 is actually a steroid hormone influencing nearly 3,000 genes in the body, including the immune system, protecting you from cancer, diabetes, heart disease, brain disorders, autoimmune disease and a host of other health problems. In fact, there is research associating over 200 diseases associated with Vitamin D deficiency. Studies have shown that Vitamin D can reduce the incidence of all cancers by over 75%.

If vitamin D is so important, why are so many people deficient in it?

Most lab reports I read from my patients, lack a vitamin D marker on them because the doctor who ordered them failed to order the test. Of those patients that do have a Vitamin D test on them, most of the vitamin D levels are well below the recommended optimal range of 50 to 70ng/ml.

One of the reasons why I believe there are so many people who are deficient in Vitamin D is because of the big scare that you hear from mainstream media that the sun is bad for you and you should stay out of it in fear of getting skin cancer. Nothing could be further from the truth. There is so much documentation and research that demonstrates the protective effect that Vitamin D has against cancer. In fact, Vitamin D by means of sunlight has a PROTECTIVE effect against skin cancer. Many of my patients have been told by their doctor to stay out of the sun in fear of getting melanoma. However, it's been shown that melanoma has been more prevalent in people who work indoors, as opposed to those who work outdoors. In addition, melanoma is often discovered in parts of the body that typically are not exposed to the sun.

I'm confused, I've always been taught that the UV rays from the sun will directly cause skin cancer. Is this true or false?

This is a loaded question. The answer to this question is really - true and false, the sun can cause cancer as well as prevent cancer. You need to use wisdom when it comes to going out in the sun. Therefore, you need to understand the difference between the harmful and beneficial rays of the sun.

Ultraviolet light comes in two forms - UVA and UVB. There is a big difference between the two of them.

UVB is the good form of ultraviolet light. When it strikes your skin, it creates a chemical reaction with the essential fatty acids and lipids on your skin and converts the sunlight into beneficial Vitamin D3 which protects you against cancer.

UVA is the bad form of ultraviolet light that penetrates deeply into your skin, creating free radical damage which CAUSES skin cancer and premature aging (wrinkles) of your skin.

UVA rays are available throughout all the hours of daylight and throughout the entire year, as opposed to UVB rays which are available only throughout certain times of the day (on average between 10AM to 3PM with the peak being around 12-1PM) and less available during certain times of the year depending upon the UVB rays or where you live. You can download the app 'D-minder,' which tells you exactly when to go out in the sun in order to capture the beneficial UVB rays. I use this app just about every day. It tells me when the sun is 35° above the horizon (which is when the UVB rays are available) and also tells you when the solar noon will occur (which is the best time to soak in the UVB rays in the shortest amount of time). I was always told that the best time to go out in the sun was earlier in the morning or later in the afternoon, but nothing could be further from the truth. The best time to go out in the sun is at solar noon which is in the middle of the day.

How much time do I need to spend in the sun to get the appropriate Vitamin D3 that I need?

This is another loaded question. There are a few factors that you need to consider. First of all, let's say you have not gone out in the sun at all because of what you were told by mainstream media, and after reading this you've realized the importance of getting regular sunlight. You don't want to make the mistake of getting too much sun too quickly. Have you ever gone on vacation or to the beach in the summer time and spent hours in the sun on the first day only to get severely sunburned? You then spent the rest of the week recuperating from making that mistake. Don't make the same mistake when it comes to getting your Vitamin D3. Start out very slowly by spending 10 minutes in the sun or when your skin starts to turn light pink and that's it. The next day, you can stay out a few minutes longer and work your way up.

If you are fair skinned, you should work your way up to 20 minutes a day, at least three times a week. It is important to note that 40% or more of your body should be exposed. The more skin that you have exposed, the less time you need to spend in the sun. It would be wise to wear a wide brimmed hat and cover your face and neck. The darker your skin is, the more time you need to spend in the sun to receive the benefits of Vitamin D3. You may need to spend 40 to 90 minutes in the sun to achieve the amount of Vitamin D3 you need if your skin is dark. Also, the more you weigh, the more time you need to spend in the sun to get adequate Vitamin D3.

If you can't spend adequate time in the sun to get your Vitamin D3, then you need to take an oral supplement of Vitamin D3 to keep your blood levels at 50 to 70 ng/ml. It's important that you use Vitamin D3 (cholecalciferol - which is the natural form of Vitamin D that your body makes when exposed to sunshine) and not vitamin D2 (ergocalciferol-which is the synthetic and inferior form of Vitamin D and 500% slower in absorption compared to Vitamin D3). Vitamin D2 is often the form of Vitamin D prescribed by your doctor and is also found in fortified foods such as pasteurized milk.

I don't understand why my Vitamin D3 levels are so low when I'm spending so much time in the sun. Why is this the case?

Occasionally, I will have a patient who claims to spend a lot of time in the sun, and yet their Vitamin D3 levels are low on their lab tests. Why is this the case? When I look at their skin color and notice that they are still on the pale side, it's because they are not exposing enough of their body to the sunlight by wearing too many clothes. When they tell me that most of their body is exposed to the sun, the next question I will ask is, "Do you wear sunscreen?" The answer is almost always, "Yes." It's impossible to get Vitamin D3 from the sunlight when you are wearing sunscreen. If my patient has a nice tan, is not wearing sunscreen, and still has low Vitamin D3 levels, I'll ask, "Do you use soap in the shower?" The answer is almost always, "Yes." It takes approximately 48 hours after you've been in the sunlight for your body to absorb the Vitamin D3 into your body. If you use soap on your body after being in the sunlight, you are washing off the oils from your skin that contains the vitamin D3, so in essence, you are washing off the Vitamin D3 that you obtained by laying out in the sun. If you are going to use soap in the shower, use it on your armpits and private areas that are typically not exposed to sunlight. It's also important to note that if you are taking medications that affect your cholesterol levels such as statin drugs, like Lipitor or proton pump inhibitors like Prilosec or Prevocid, you run the risk of having lower Vitamin D3 levels, as you need cholesterol to transport Vitamin D3 which is a steroid hormone in the body. These medications can also affect the transport and function of other hormones in the body.

In summary: Vitamin D3 is actually a steroid hormone influencing nearly 3,000 genes in the body, including the immune system protecting you from cancer, diabetes, heart disease, brain disorders, autoimmune disease and a host of other health problems. In fact, there is research associating over 200 diseases associated with Vitamin D deficiency, and studies have shown that Vitamin D can reduce the incidence of all cancers by over 75%. Most people are deficient in Vitamin D3 because they have been told that the sun is harmful, causing skin cancer, but what they fail to understand is that the sun produces two types of ultraviolet rays: UVA (the harmful rays that cause skin cancer, destroys Vitamin D3 and causes wrinkles) and UVB (the beneficial rays that cause your body to produce Vitamin D3 protecting you from cancer, including skin cancer). The UVB rays are accessible only during certain times of the day and year when the sun is 35° above the horizon. The app 'D-minder' lets you know exactly when these rays are available, including the best time to obtain Vitamin D3 which is at solar noon. There are many factors influencing Vitamin D3 absorption, including skin color, amount of skin exposure, and even bathing practices. Keeping your Vitamin D3 levels at 50 to 70 ng/ml is essential to staying healthy.

"I am a board certified family medicine doctor who specializes in integrative wellness medicine. When I injured my left shoulder from playing beach volleyball, I was recommended to see Dr. Taylor. Dr Taylor performed a focused yet thorough history and examination. He helped me identify possible triggers for my pain, including some dietary foods and EMF from my Fit Bit device. After completing 6 treatments on my left shoulder and left upper back, I no longer had any pain, I regained my normal range of motion, and was able to play beach volleyball without any restrictions. I feel Dr. Taylor has a comprehensive approach to assist anyone with pain."
~Dr. Marcela Dominguez, M.D

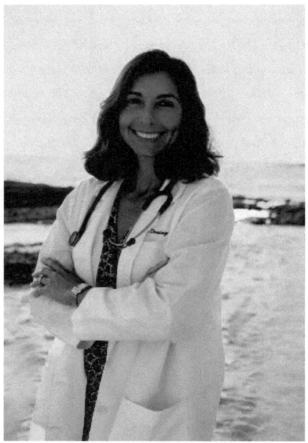

(Dr. Marcela Dominguez, M.D.)

Chapter 10

Bottom Line:
Make That Change Today,
For A Better You Tomorrow

Strength does not come from winning.
Your struggles develop your strengths.
When you go through hardships and decide not to surrender,
that is strength."
~Arnold Schwarzenegger

When one door closes, another opens;
but we often look so long and so regretfully
upon the closed door
that we do not see the one which has opened for us.
~Alexander Graham Bell

Over the past 25 years, patients come into my office with some type of symptom, health challenge, or pain. I try to explain to them that whenever their body manifests with a symptom, it's trying to tell them that there is an imbalance somewhere and it needs to be corrected before something worse happens.

Symptoms are your friends that are trying to warn you about a problem you have. Although they may be uncomfortable and inconvenient, you can be thankful that you have a warning signal to make a change in your lifestyle or daily habits. Contrast that with the person who has a heart problem and the first symptom they experience is a sudden-death heart attack. This occurs in about 30% of patients who have heart disease. They have no opportunity to make a lifestyle change. They never had any warnings that they had a problem.

What you do without warning is critical for your longevity and overall health.

The problem is typically caused by stress. Once the stress has been corrected, you must continue to work on eliminating or minimizing the stressors in your lifestyle that led to your pain in the first place, while at the same time adding or maintaining the actions you took to get out of pain.

In other words, it goes back to the bank account illustration. You must minimize the withdrawals in your health checking account and maximize the deposits at the same time. Your daily habits will play a big factor in whether or not the symptoms stay away and you maintain good health.

So, let's look again at the three stressors that influence pain.

Physical Stressors: Let's start by breaking down your day. In chapter 6, I gave you specific information to help you sleep better. Follow those instructions for a better night's sleep. Eight hours off the bat are invested in sleeping. Therefore, it's imperative that you have a supportive bed to offer you your best night's sleep. If a third of your life is spent sleeping, it makes sense to invest in a bed that will properly support your spine and body. In addition, it's important to have a bed made with non-toxic materials so you're not breathing in toxins all night while you're sleeping. I recommend the company, Sleep Level. Their bed adjusts to your spine no matter what your weight is and it is chiropractic-approved. Sleep Level gives you 90 days to try it out, and if you don't like it they will pick it up from you. I have spoken with my Sleep Level representative and asked them if they would give you a discount because you have read this book, and they agreed. Just mention my account number xxx and they will give you 10% off your order.

Another third of your day is most likely spent sitting. This needs to change. Make every effort to sit less and to convert your workstation into a standup desk like I mentioned in Chapter 8. Sitting is the new smoking, as mentioned in this chapter and you're going to be much healthier with less sitting.

Another third of your day is most likely spent standing. The shoes you wear are imperative for proper support and health to your lower back. This is a really difficult problem for most people because, let's face it, we're all a slave to fashion and we want to look good. Sorry ladies, but wearing shoes with a heel will create tension in the lower back. The higher the heel, the more the tension. We were not meant to walk around in heels. Wearing a heel will shorten the Achilles tendon, alter the proprioceptive function in your feet, and create poor balance for the body. I can prove it to you right now. Find another person to help you prove my point. Stand on the floor barefoot. Bend your elbows at a 90° angle with your elbows at your side. Make a fist with your left hand and place it on top of your right hand. Now have someone push down on the fist of your left hand and notice how stable you are. Do the same thing while barefoot but raise both heels up slightly to the level where they're raised when you're wearing your shoes and perform the same test. You'll notice immediately how unstable you are when the person pushes down on your left fist. Now I realize for many of you, knowing this information isn't going to change your mind about the shoes you wear. I have no problem with that as long as you perform this exercise I'm going to give you to counteract the stressors of wearing heels.

Here it is: Look at the shoes you wear often and measure the height of the heel. Now grab a book that's about as thick as the heel height of your shoe. Place the balls of your bare feet on the book (you can also use a 2 x 4 board if that's the height of your heels in your shoes) to stretch out the Achilles tendon. I have a formula you can use for the amount of time to perform this stretch. For every hour you've been wearing that shoe you need to stretch your Achilles for one minute. In other words if you're on your feet for 8 hours in heeled shoes, then you need to stretch that Achilles tendon for 8 minutes. Some of you may be thinking you don't have time to spend 8 minutes stretching out your Achilles tendon every day. To make it easy you can do this stretch throughout the day while you're at work even for 1 minute while performing other tasks. Or you can do it at the end of the day when you get home and are preparing dinner or while you're watching TV at night.

Another main source of stress many people aren't aware of is how the exercises they're doing on a regular basis are affecting their body. Chapter 7 goes into detail about the exercises you can do to get out of pain and to live long. Follow those instructions and see the difference it makes in your life.

Chemical Stressors: Identifying which foods are creating inflammation and pain in your body is vital to removing your pain. You can go to the greatest chiropractor in the world, do the best exercises known to humans that are perfect for your body type, and still have pain because you're eating foods that are creating inflammation and pain. Chapter 3 goes into this with great detail. Chapter 5 talks about the importance of water and hydration.

Emotional/Mental Stressors: This is probably one of the most challenging stressors to manage and eliminate on a regular basis because people just don't like dealing with their emotions. They often deny them, sweep them under the rug, push them off to the side, and don't have the time, energy, or desire to manage their emotions. It's important to set aside time each day to reflect, think about, and process your emotions so they don't become a source of pain for you. Don't spend your entire day in the presence of people while constantly interacting and communicating. You need time for yourself. This is one of the simplest ways of staying healthy and pain-free as discussed in Chapter 4, but is often the most neglected. Make it a habit to process your emotions instead of stuffing them and you'll see the benefits of being more balanced and having less pain.

I would like to leave you with one final thought. Two of the most powerful words in the financial world are "Compound Interest." Compound Interest is so powerful because it has a snowball effect where your money is making money for you. It's financial momentum that's gained and accumulated over time. It can make the poor become rich and the wealthy become wealthier. Albert Einstein said, "Compound Interest is the eighth wonder of the world. He who understands it, earns it...he who doesn't...pays it."

Did you get that? "He who understands it, earns it...he who doesn't...pays it." What does Compound Interest have to do with your health? Everything! Every day I see people who either have Compound Interest working for them or against them. What do I mean by that? When Compound Interest is working against you, you've accumulated so much stress in your life that it actually starts to affect, not just one area of your health, but many areas. It's like having credit card debt when your interest rate is 18%. When this happens, you're in trouble. You're going to crash sooner or later. It's just a matter of time. You're in so much debt in your health account that even a large payment doesn't seem to make a dent.

I see this in my practice all the time. Let me to explain what I'm talking about. A patient comes in with pain that's so bad, even the slightest amount of pressure elicits a pain that feels unbearable. They can't sleep, they can't think straight, they're in a grouchy mood all the time, they're unproductive at work, and they're useless to others at home because all they can focus on is their pain. They may have been taking medication for years which has caused more inflammation in their large intestine and toxicity in their liver and kidneys. These organs are stressed and are referring pain to other parts of the body as well. As a result of not being themselves, they have strained the relationships around them and are in emotional locks because they have anxiety, resentment, anger, and bitterness bound up inside them for obvious reasons. No one around them understands them. With these patients, even the slightest movement or setback can send them in a tailspin for weeks. Compound Interest is working against them.

On the flip side of the coin, you can have Compound Interest working for you. In other words, those patients who are constantly working on reducing their physical, chemical, and emotional stressors and are placing deposits in their health account are feeling healthy, strong, alert, energetic, and with no pain or symptoms at all. When these patients have stressors that unexpectedly come upon them, the stressor may or may not cause pain, and if it does, the pain isn't there for long. They heal quickly and bounce back rapidly from setbacks because they have Compound Interest working for them.

I recently had a patient with symptoms that were so bad, she didn't think they'd ever go away. They were from a pain she had in her legs and back for decades. She got on a program to eliminate the stressors in her body, started implementing lifestyle changes, and her symptoms slowly started to disappear. Ultimately the pain completely disappeared. She continues to invest in her health for maintenance by visiting me once per month and feels better than ever. Her back no longer bothers her, she sleeps like a baby, she pops up out of bed in the morning with vigor and vitality, and she's able to handle stress with ease. Her investment slowly, over time, began to make big changes in her health and she went from having Compound Interest working against her to now having it work for her.

You must remember this: SLOW AND STEADY WINS THE RACE. 'Perseverance' triumphs over 'quick and easy' every day of the week. Start investing in your health today and you'll see that over time, you'll have Compound Interest working for you and not against you. If you move in this direction, you'll have no regrets about making an investment in your health—which is one of the greatest investments you can make! You see, when you start to invest in your health, you not only improve the quality of your life, but you also start to positively affect the lives of your family and loved ones. Do you want to see your loved ones get healthier?

Great! One of the ways this happens is when YOU start to get healthier yourself.

I've seen this time and again in my practice. One family member takes their health to a new level and it often raises the entire family's level of health. It starts with one person: who will it be?

How about if it starts with you? Why not take the principles you've learned in this book and start applying them to your life TODAY! Imagine waking up with no pain, feeling energetic, being able to do what you love doing, and enjoying life to the fullest. If others have been able to get rid of pain they thought they would have to live with for the rest of their life, why can't you get rid of yours?

I believe you can and I hope this book will help you accomplish your dreams and goals.

Mark Twain once said, "The secret of getting ahead is getting started."

Start today for a healthier you tomorrow. I wish you all the best!

7 Habits to Experience Pain Free Living!

Made in USA - Kendallville, IN
1174300_9781546479109